From "Stress Septal Sign" to Global "Heart Remodeling"

From "Stress Septal Sign" to Global "Heart Remodeling"

Editors

Mario J. Garcia
Fatih Yalcin

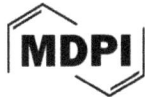

Basel • Beijing • Wuhan • Barcelona • Belgrade • Novi Sad • Cluj • Manchester

Editors
Mario J. Garcia
Montefiore Medical Center
Bronx, NY
USA

Fatih Yalcin
UCSF HEALTH
San Francisco, CA
USA

Editorial Office
MDPI AG
Grosspeteranlage 5
4052 Basel, Switzerland

This is a reprint of articles from the Special Issue published online in the open access journal *Journal of Clinical Medicine* (ISSN 2077-0383) (available at: https://www.mdpi.com/journal/jcm/special_issues/clinical_frontiers_heart_failure).

For citation purposes, cite each article independently as indicated on the article page online and as indicated below:

Lastname, A.A.; Lastname, B.B. Article Title. *Journal Name* **Year**, *Volume Number*, Page Range.

ISBN 978-3-7258-1845-7 (Hbk)
ISBN 978-3-7258-1846-4 (PDF)
doi.org/10.3390/books978-3-7258-1846-4

Cover image courtesy of Prof. Dr. Fatih Yalcin

© 2024 by the authors. Articles in this book are Open Access and distributed under the Creative Commons Attribution (CC BY) license. The book as a whole is distributed by MDPI under the terms and conditions of the Creative Commons Attribution-NonCommercial-NoDerivs (CC BY-NC-ND) license.

Contents

Preface vii

Fatih Yalcin and Mario J. Garcia
It Is Time to Focus on "Segmental Remodeling" with Validated Biomarkers as "Stressed Heart Morphology" in Prevention of Heart Failure
Reprinted from: *J. Clin. Med.* **2022**, *11*, 4180, doi:10.3390/jcm11144180 1

Elena Medvedeva, Lyudmila Korostovtseva, Mihail Bochkarev, Anastasiya Shumeiko, Aelita Berezina, Maria Simonenko, et al.
The Prognostic Role of Polysomnography Parameters in Heart Failure Patients with Previous Decompensation
Reprinted from: *J. Clin. Med.* **2022**, *11*, 3656, doi:10.3390/jcm11133656 3

Frank A. Flachskampf and Tomasz Baron
The Role of Novel Cardiac Imaging for Contemporary Management of Heart Failure
Reprinted from: *J. Clin. Med.* **2022**, *11*, 6201, doi:10.3390/jcm11206201 14

Andrzej Osiecki, Wacław Kochman, Klaus K. Witte, Małgorzata Mańczak, Robert Olszewski and Dariusz Michałkiewicz
Cardiomyopathy Associated with Right Ventricular Apical Pacing-Systematic Review and Meta-Analysis
Reprinted from: *J. Clin. Med.* **2022**, *11*, 6889, doi:10.3390/jcm11236889 29

Luminita Iliuta, Andreea Gabriella Andronesi, Eugenia Panaitescu, Madalina Elena Rac-Albu, Alexandru Scafa-Udriște and Horațiu Moldovan
Challenges for Management of Dilated Cardiomyopathy during COVID-19 Pandemic—A Telemedicine Application
Reprinted from: *J. Clin. Med.* **2022**, *11*, 7411, doi:10.3390/jcm11247411 42

Ivona Mustapic, Darija Bakovic, Zora Susilovic Grabovac and Josip A Borovac
Impact of SGLT2 Inhibitor Therapy on Right Ventricular Function in Patients with Heart Failure and Reduced Ejection Fraction
Reprinted from: *J. Clin. Med.* **2023**, *12*, 42, doi:10.3390/jcm12010042 56

Teruhiko Imamura, Toshihide Izumida, Nikhil Narang, Hiroshi Onoda, Masaki Nakagaito, Shuhei Tanaka, et al.
Association between Remote Dielectric Sensing and Estimated Plasma Volume to Assess Body Fluid Distribution
Reprinted from: *J. Clin. Med.* **2023**, *12*, 463, doi:10.3390/jcm12020463 71

Emel Celiker Guler, Mehmet Onur Omaygenc, Deniz Dilan Naki, Arzu Yazar, Ibrahim Oguz Karaca and Esin Korkut
Isolated Subclinical Right Ventricle Systolic Dysfunction in Patients after Liver Transplantation
Reprinted from: *J. Clin. Med.* **2023**, *12*, 2289, doi:10.3390/jcm12062289 79

Magdalena Dudek, Marta Kałużna-Oleksy, Jacek Migaj, Filip Sawczak, Helena Krysztofiak, Maciej Lesiak and Ewa Straburzyńska-Migaj
sST2 and Heart Failure—Clinical Utility and Prognosis
Reprinted from: *J. Clin. Med.* **2023**, *12*, 3136, doi:10.3390/jcm12093136 89

Łukasz Wołowiec, Joanna Banach, Jacek Budzyński, Anna Wołowiec, Mariusz Kozakiewicz, Maciej Bieliński, et al.
Prognostic Value of Plasma Catestatin Concentration in Patients with Heart Failure with Reduced Ejection Fraction in Two-Year Follow-Up
Reprinted from: *J. Clin. Med.* **2023**, *12*, 4208, doi:10.3390/jcm12134208 . . . . **101**

Fatih Yalçin, Maria Roselle Abraham and Mario J. Garcia
Stress and Heart in Remodeling Process: Multiple Stressors at the Same Time Kill
Reprinted from: *J. Clin. Med.* **2024**, *13*, 2597, doi:10.3390/jcm13092597 . . . . **116**

Preface

This work is sufficient to inform the readers of the importance of early biomarkers and management in heart failure.

Unfortunately, the medical device industry is prioritizing advanced-stage treatments by neglecting biomarkers. Targeting and treating advanced-stage diseases is not only not cost-effective, but it is less effective than the making significant efforts during early stages of disease.

Mario J. Garcia is my mentor and research partner, and he has been conducting research into the crucial role of early management in cardiology since beginning of the century.

As the Editor, I believe that we cannot better predict heart problems in the global population if we do not increase the number of relevant scientific products available.

We thank to Judy Li for her support and MDPI to allowing us to produce this work.

Mario J. Garcia and Fatih Yalcin
Editors

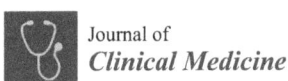

Editorial

It Is Time to Focus on "Segmental Remodeling" with Validated Biomarkers as "Stressed Heart Morphology" in Prevention of Heart Failure

Fatih Yalcin [1,*] and Mario J. Garcia [2,3]

1 Department of Cardiology, UCSF HEALTH, School of Medicine, Cardiac Imaging, San Francisco, CA 94143, USA
2 Cardiology Division, Montefiore Medical Center, Bronx, NY 10461, USA; mariogar@montefiore.org
3 Albert Einstein College of Medicine, Bronx, NY 10461, USA
* Correspondence: fyhopkins@gmail.com

Citation: Yalcin, F.; Garcia, M.J. It Is Time to Focus on "Segmental Remodeling" with Validated Biomarkers as "Stressed Heart Morphology" in Prevention of Heart Failure. *J. Clin. Med.* **2022**, *11*, 4180. https://doi.org/10.3390/jcm11144180

Received: 4 July 2022
Accepted: 14 July 2022
Published: 19 July 2022

Publisher's Note: MDPI stays neutral with regard to jurisdictional claims in published maps and institutional affiliations.

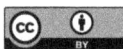

Copyright: © 2022 by the authors. Licensee MDPI, Basel, Switzerland. This article is an open access article distributed under the terms and conditions of the Creative Commons Attribution (CC BY) license (https://creativecommons.org/licenses/by/4.0/).

In cardiovascular medicine, hemodynamic stress with hypertension is a major risk. Recently, we have invented a new segmental paradigm for left ventricular (LV) remodeling by describing microscopic remodeling for the first time and started to mention the blood pressure fluctuations on initial remodeling, namely, basal septal hypertrophy (BSH) [1–3]. Adaptation to hemodynamic stress is a long-standing process, which we validated this remodeling phase in small animals using third-generation microscopic ultrasonography [4,5]. The remodeling process starts on the septal base, which continues for almost half of the course and progresses quite regularly over the midapical segment. This first period is associated with increased tissue dynamics, detected by tissue Doppler, and increased fluid dynamics [6,7].

Therefore, we have called this period the adaptive phase of LV remodeling and validated BSH as an early imaging biomarker. We previously reported that BSH represents exercise hypertension and increased rate-pressure product at stress in human hypertension [8]. Interestingly, we realized that there is a huge difference in morphology between human and animal BSH morphology after our validation studies [1]. Thus, we have reported the remarkable details of these morphological differences over septal base [1]. Naturally, irregularity and heterogeneity in human beings have been implemented to cognitive function, and recently, our initial data have been exhibited at ESH 2022 [9].

Furthermore, the most important aspect of our animal validation data on microscopic remodeling is that the LV base represents the specific location for a variety of stress stimuli and could be described as the "Stressed Heart Morphology". In fact, we have pointed out not only a functional mechanism due to increased afterload in hypertension, but emotional and mechanic mechanisms in acute stress cardiomyopathy and aortic stenosis, respectively [10–13]. Increased sympathetic drive, independent from acute or chronic pathogenesis, using BSH as the early imaging biomarker in diagnoses of SHM, and effective medical management in a timely fashion, can contribute to the prevention of heart failure.

Despite scientific developments from real-time three-dimensional segmental volume analysis at Cleveland Clinic [14] to the animal validation studies by third-generation microscopic ultrasound at Johns Hopkins [4,5], and then microscopic remodeling using comparisons of human and animal data at UCSF [1–3] over two decades, we still do not know the certain prevalence and potential role of LV segmental remodeling and early imaging biomarkers in populations who face daily fluctuations of extremely dangerous hemodynamic stress.

The global absence of segmental data, beyond cross-sectional measurements regarding cardiac structures, and the absence of hemodynamic data under stress in individuals with incidentally detected BSH, could possibly result in underestimations of the relationship between hemodynamic overload and septal remodeling. Moreover, we have recently suggested that the discrepancy between predominant BSH in adaptation to stress stimuli and thinner midapical segment could be important in the progression to heart failure and increased mortality [12].

In conclusion, SHM represents the morphologic and functional discrepancy of LV segments. The current report emphasizes that incidentally detected early imaging biomarkers may be beneficial and could be used widely to avoid increased numbers of cardiac pathologies with LV remodeling and previously undiagnosed heart failure cases.

Please consider contributing to this issue, since segmental assessment of remodeling is a promising approach for prediction of advanced LV remodeling and presumably increased mortality. Your contribution will support "THE POOL DATA OF SEGMENTAL REMODELING" in the near future.

Funding: F.Y. is supported by the U.S. Government Fulbright Scholarship, Washington DC, USA, and serves as an Editor for a Special Issue on Heart Failure. (https://www.mdpi.com/journal/jcm/special_issues/clinical_frontiers_heart_failure, accessed on 3 July 2022).

Conflicts of Interest: The authors declare no conflict of interest.

References

1. Yalçin, F.; Yalçin, H.; Küçükler, N.; Arslan, S.; Akkuş, O.; Kurtul, A.; Abraham, M.R. Basal septal hypertrophy as the early imaging biomarker for adaptive phase of remodeling prior to heart failure. *J. Clin. Med.* **2022**, *11*, 75. [CrossRef] [PubMed]
2. Yalçin, F.; Yalçin, H.; Abraham, M.R.; Abraham, T.P. Hemodynamic stress and microscopic remodeling. *Int. J. Cardiol. Cardiovasc. Risk Prev.* **2021**, *11*, 200115. [CrossRef] [PubMed]
3. Yalçin, F.; Yalçin, H.; Abraham, T.P. Exercise hypertension should be recalled in basal septal hypertrophy as the early imaging biomarker in patients with stressed heart morphology. *Blood Press Monit.* **2020**, *25*, 118–119. [CrossRef] [PubMed]
4. Yalçin, F.; Kucukler, N.; Cingolani, O.; Mbiyangandu, B.; Sorensen, L.; Pinherio, A.; Abraham, M.R.; Abraham, T.P. Evolution of ventricular hypertrophy and myocardial mechanics in physiologic and pathologic hypertrophy. *J. Appl. Physiol.* **2019**, *126*, 354–362. [CrossRef] [PubMed]
5. Yalçin, F.; Kucukler, N.; Cingolani, O.; Mbiyangandu, B.; Sorensen, L.L.; Pinheiro, A.C.; Abraham, M.R.; Abraham, T.P. Intracavitary gradient in mice with early regional remodeling at the compensatory hyperactive stage prior to left ventricular tissue dysfunction. *J. Am. Coll. Cardiol.* **2020**, *75*, 1585. [CrossRef]
6. Yalçin, F.; Yalçin, H.; Abraham, M.R.; Abraham, T.P. Ultimate phases of hypertensive heart disease and stressed heart morphology by conventional and novel cardiac imaging. *Am. J. Cardiovasc. Dis.* **2021**, *11*, 628–634. [PubMed]
7. Yalçin, F.; Abraham, M.R.; Abraham, T.P. Basal septal hypertrophy: Extremely sensitive region to variety of stress stimuli and stressed heart morphology. *J. Hypertens.* **2022**, *40*, 626–627. [CrossRef] [PubMed]
8. Yalçin, F.; Yigit, F.; Erol, T.; Baltali, M.; E Korkmaz, M.; Müderrisoğlu, H. Effect of dobutamine stress on basal septal tissue dynamics in hypertensive patients with basal septal hypertrophy. *J. Hum. Hypertens.* **2006**, *20*, 628–630. [CrossRef] [PubMed]
9. Yalçin, F.; Melek, I.; Mutlu, T. Stressed heart morphology and neurologic stress score effect beyond hemodynamic stress on focal geometry. *J. Hypertens.* **2022**, *40* (Suppl. S1), e79. [CrossRef]
10. Yalçin, F.; Müderrisoğlu, H. Tako-tsubo cardiomyopathy may be associated with cardiac geometric features as observed in hypetensive heart disease. *Int. J. Cardiol.* **2009**, *135*, 251–252. [CrossRef] [PubMed]
11. Yalçin, F.; Yalçin, H.; Abraham, T. Stress-induced regional features of left ventricle is related to pathogenesis of clinical conditions with both acute and chronic stress. *Int. J. Cardiol.* **2010**, *145*, 367–368. [CrossRef] [PubMed]
12. Yalçin, F.; Abraham, R.; Abraham, T.P. Myocardial aspects in aortic stenosis and functional increased afterload conditions in patients with stressed heart morphology. *Ann. Thorac. Cardiovasc. Surg.* **2021**, *27*, 332–334. [CrossRef] [PubMed]
13. Yalçin, F.; Abraham, M.R.; Abraham, T.P. It is time to assess left ventricular segmental remodeling in aortic stenosis. *Eur. Heart J. Cardiovasc. Imaging* **2022**, jeac071. [CrossRef] [PubMed]
14. Yalçin, F.; Shiota, T.; Odabashian, J.; Agler, D.; Greenberg, N.L.; Garcia, M.J.; Lever, H.M.; Thomas, J.D. Comparison by realtime three-dimensional echocardiography of left ventricular geometry in hypertrophic cardiomyopathy versus secondary left ventricular hypertrophy. *Am. J. Cardiol.* **2000**, *85*, 1035–1038. [CrossRef]

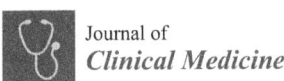

Article

The Prognostic Role of Polysomnography Parameters in Heart Failure Patients with Previous Decompensation

Elena Medvedeva *, Lyudmila Korostovtseva, Mihail Bochkarev, Anastasiya Shumeiko, Aelita Berezina, Maria Simonenko, Yulia Sazonova, Andrey Kozlenok and Yurii Sviryaev

Almazov National Medical Research Centre, 197341 St. Petersburg, Russia; lyudmila_korosto@mail.ru (L.K.); michail_bv@list.ru (M.B.); nastya0594@mail.ru (A.S.); berezina_av@almazovcentre.ru (A.B.); ladymaria.dr@gmail.com (M.S.); yulia.via.sazonova@gmail.com (Y.S.); kozlenok_av@almazovcentre.ru (A.K.); yusvyr@yandex.ru (Y.S.)
* Correspondence: elenamedvedeva544@gmail.com; Tel.: +7-931-963-28-78

Citation: Medvedeva, E.; Korostovtseva, L.; Bochkarev, M.; Shumeiko, A.; Berezina, A.; Simonenko, M.; Sazonova, Y.; Kozlenok, A.; Sviryaev, Y. The Prognostic Role of Polysomnography Parameters in Heart Failure Patients with Previous Decompensation. *J. Clin. Med.* 2022, 11, 3656. https://doi.org/10.3390/jcm11133656

Academic Editor: Alessandro Delitala

Received: 18 May 2022
Accepted: 21 June 2022
Published: 24 June 2022

Publisher's Note: MDPI stays neutral with regard to jurisdictional claims in published maps and institutional affiliations.

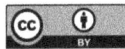

Copyright: © 2022 by the authors. Licensee MDPI, Basel, Switzerland. This article is an open access article distributed under the terms and conditions of the Creative Commons Attribution (CC BY) license (https://creativecommons.org/licenses/by/4.0/).

Abstract: Background: Sleep-disordered breathing (SDB) is a widespread comorbidity in patients with chronic heart failure (HF) and may have a deleterious effect on the pathogenesis of HF. We aimed to evaluate the prognostic role of polysomnography parameters in HF patients with previous decompensation. Methods: 123 patients were included in the prospective cohort study. In addition to the standard examination, all patients underwent polysomnography (PSG). Results: The Kaplan–Meier analysis showed the incidence of the combined endpoint differs between LVEF categories $\leq 25.5\%$ vs. $>25.5\%$ ($\chi^2 = 9.6$, log rank $p = 0.002$), NTpro-BNP > 680 vs. ≤ 680 pg/mL ($\chi^2 = 12.7$, log rank $p = 0.001$), VO$_2$peak categories <16 vs. ≥ 16 mL/min/kg ($\chi^2 = 14.2$, log rank $p = 0.001$), VE/VCO$_2$ slope ≥ 38.5 vs. <38.5 ($\chi^2 = 14.5$, log rank $p = 0.001$), wake after sleep onset >40 min vs. ≤ 40 min ($\chi^2 = 9.7$, log rank $p = 0.03$), and sleep stage 2 (S$_2$) <44% vs. $\geq 44\%$ ($\chi^2 = 12.4$, log rank $p = 0.001$). Conclusion: Among the PSG parameters, WASO > 40 min and S$_2$ < 44% were associated with a combined endpoint in patients with previous decompensation of HF. Moreover, higher NT-proBNP and VE/VCO$_2$ slope, lower LVEF, and VO$_{2peak}$ were also independent factors of a poor prognosis.

Keywords: heart failure; sleep apnea; prognosis; polysomnography; wake after sleep onset

1. Introduction

Sleep-disordered breathing (SDB) is associated with more frequent readmissions and worse outcomes in patients with heart failure (HF) [1–3]. According to several studies, sleep apnea in patients with HF is associated with an increased frequency of life-threatening arrhythmias during night hours, confirmed by an increased frequency of nocturnal shocks from implantable cardioverter–defibrillators [4].

While obstructive sleep apnea (OSA) is shown to be an independent risk factor for the development of HF and a worse prognosis [5], central sleep apnea (CSA) is possibly a marker of HF severity, with increased neurohumoral activation, increased pulmonary capillary wedge pressure, and worsening HF [6]. The sympathetic activation that occurs in patients with CSA might adversely affect the prognosis in HF patients. The sympathetic activation is associated with the incidence of apneas, frequency, and severity of hypoxia through chemoreflex activation. This mechanism suggests that CSA can play a crucial role in the worsening of the left ventricular function and clinical status of HF patients, emphasizing the existence of a bidirectional relationship between CSA and HF [1].

The severity of apnea is usually assessed using the apnea–hypopnea index, but this index, associated with prognosis, probably does not reflect all the complex pathophysiological mechanisms that can lead to adverse outcomes in heart failure. Moreover, the prognostic value of the parameters characterizing the structure and quality of sleep in HF patients is still uncertain.

Episodes of decompensation of HF worsen the prognosis and exacerbate comorbid conditions. In the present study, we aim to evaluate the clinical features and the prognostic role of polysomnography parameters in HF patients with previous decompensation.

2. Materials and Methods

2.1. Patients and Study Design

In a prospective cohort study, we enrolled patients who were eligible according to the following inclusion criteria: patients with chronic heart failure II-IV functional class NYHA, 18–74 years old, and hospitalized with decompensation of HF.

Exclusion criteria were inability to participate or consent, acute coronary syndrome or recent stroke (within 90 days of admission), severe chronic obstructive pulmonary disease (COPD) with forced expiratory volume in 1 s (FEV1) less than 50%, and oxygen therapy.

All patients underwent standard clinical examination after compensation, a 6 min walking test, 12-lead electrocardiography, transthoracic echocardiography, polysomnography, cardiopulmonary exercise testing, and venous blood sampling. All examinations were performed before discharge in patients without significant congestion, if possible, and while sleeping in a horizontal position. The main characteristics of the patients are presented in Table 1.

Table 1. Baseline characteristics of the cohort.

Parameter	Baseline
Age, years	55 (46–60)
Male/female, n	103/20
Body mass index, kg/m^2	26.13 (22.2–32.75)
NYHA functional class, n	
II	46
III	52
IV	25
Left ventricle ejection fraction (LVEF), %	27 (21–32.5)
Reduced LVEF (<40%), n	108
Midrange LVEF (40–49%), n	10
Preserved LVEF (>50%), n	5
HF etiology	n
Coronary artery disease (CAD), n	73
Non-CAD, n	50
Dilated cardiomyopathy	44
Restrictive cardiomyopathy	1
Hypertrophic cardiomyopathy	1
Arrhythmogenic dysplasia of the right ventricle	2
Non-compaction cardiomyopathy	2
Comorbid conditions	n
Diabetes mellitus, n	89
Obesity, n	81
Anemia, n	43
Atrial fibrillation, n	49
Smoking status	
Current or ex-smoker, n	76
Nonsmoker, n	47
Concomitant medications and devices	n (%)
Beta-blockers	114 (93)
Angiotensin converting enzyme inhibitors	75 (61)
Angiotensin receptor blockers	30 (24)
Valsartan + sacubitril	5 (4)
Mineralocorticoid receptor antagonists	97 (79)
Diuretics	89 (72)
Anticoagulants	57 (46)
Acetylsalicylic acid	80 (65)
Nitrates	42 (34)
CRT-D	12 (10)

CAD—coronary artery disease, CRT-D—cardiac resynchronization treatment with defibrillator, LVEF—left ventricular ejection fraction. Values are indicated as number of patients n (%) or median (1st and 3rd quartiles).

The study protocol was approved by the ethics committee. All participants signed written informed consent.

2.2. Methods

2.2.1. Polysomnography

After compensation, the patients underwent in-lab polysomnography (PSG) (Embla N7000, Natus, Middleton, WI, USA). If patients needed constant monitoring, a portable recording system was used to perform PSG in heart failure units (MiniScreen Pro, Löwenstein Medical, Hamburg, Germany). PSG was repeated in patients who underwent heart transplantation (HTx) during follow-up (usually 6 months after transplantation).

PSG analysis was manually performed by two experienced investigators using custom software. Episodes of apnea–hypopnea were assessed according to the guidelines of the American Academy of Sleep Medicine Task Force [7]. Based on the apnea–hypopnea index (AHI), sleep apnea was defined as none (AHI < 5/h), mild (AHI 5–14.9/h), moderate (AHI 15–29.9/h), or severe (AHI $\geq$ 30/h). We also estimated the following indicators: total sleep time (TST), duration of sleep stages (S_1, S_2, S_3, REM), WASO (wake after sleep onset), sleep efficiency, oxygen desaturation index (ODI), average and minimum saturation O_2, and the maximum and mean duration of apnea.

2.2.2. Echocardiographic Examination

All patients underwent complete transthoracic echocardiographic studies with a Vivid 7 (GE Vingmed Ultrasound AS, Horten, Norway) system. Two-dimensional-mode (2Dmode), M-mode echocardiography, and tissue Doppler imaging were conducted. Three consecutive cycles were averaged for every parameter. The guidelines and expert consensus for echocardiographic cardiac chamber quantification were used for further imaging analysis [8,9].

2.2.3. Cardiopulmonary Exercise Testing

Cardiopulmonary exercise testing (CPET) was conducted using the breath-by-breath method on an ergospirometer, Oxycon Pro (Cardinal Health, Norderstedt, Germany). Patients performed symptom-limited, continuously increasing physical activity (RAMP protocol) on a bicycle ergometer with a load increment of 10 W/min. The subjective sensations of the patients were evaluated on a 10-point Borg scale.

Criteria for test termination consisted of the following: achievement of the maximum possible physical load for the individual or listed conditions, significant chest pain, ischemic changes in the ECG (ST segment depression > 2.0 mm; T wave inversion; new Q wave), decrease in blood pressure, sustained supraventricular or ventricular tachycardia, presyncope, syncope, unbearable dyspnea, disorientation, and loss of coordination.

The following test parameters were evaluated: peak oxygen consumption (VO_2peak), anaerobic threshold level, heart rate increase (HR) during testing (HR/VO_2 slope), HR reserve (the difference between the predicted HR max and HR max achieved during testing), the oxygen pulse (VO_2/HR), and the ventilator equivalent of CO_2 (VE/VCO_2 slope). The value of VO_2peak or VO_2max $\geq$ 85% of the proper value and the level of anaerobic threshold corresponding to 40–60% of VO_2max were considered normal.

2.2.4. Blood Analysis and BIOMARKERS

Blood samples were collected one week after compensation. The following blood tests were conducted: complete blood count, electrolytes, blood chemistry, lipid profile values, and serum protein. The glomerular filtration rate (GFR) was calculated by the CKD-EPI equation.

The plasma levels of the N-terminal prohormone of brain natriuretic peptide (NT-proBNP) and soluble form of suppression of tumorigenicity-2 (sST2) were measured after compensation using the enzyme immunoassay technique (ELISA kit), according to the instructions of the manufacturer.

2.2.5. Follow-Up

The individuals were followed up with for a maximum of 9.14 years. The collection of information about adverse events was carried out twice a year and provided by patients via telephone calls. Other status reports and information about the time and cause of death were obtained from various sources, including relatives, general practitioners, hospitals, and local registration offices.

The combined endpoint included the first event of death from any cause, left ventricular assistant device (LVAD) implantation, HTx, non-fatal myocardial infarction, repeat revascularization, and stroke. Death was considered a priority event, and the time of occurrence of the event was regarded as the time of death.

During follow-up, patient management was conducted according to discretion of the treating physician based on the European Society of Cardiology guidelines.

2.2.6. Statistical Methods

Continuous variables were presented as mean± standard deviation or median (quartile 1–quartile 3) for skewed distributions. Categorical variables were mentioned as frequencies in percent. For testing the hypotheses, 2-sided alternatives were analyzed, and the type I error rate was 5%. Due to the abnormality of the distribution, the Mann–Whitney test was used to compare independent samples, and Fisher's exact test was used for comparing categorical variables.

To investigate the predictive abilities of different parameters, a ROC curve analysis was constructed. Survival analysis was carried out using Kaplan–Meier curves. Log rank tests were used to compare survival between the different groups. All analyses were conducted in IBM SPSS Statistics version 25.0.

3. Results

3.1. HF Population

All patient characteristics are described in Table 1. Coronary artery disease was present in 58.7% of patients. The median of left ventricular ejection fraction (LVEF) was 27.0%, and only 8.3% of patients had HF with preserved EF.

3.2. Prognosis

According to follow-up data, 76 patients reached the combined endpoint. The distribution by clinical, laboratory, and instrumental parameters is presented in Table 2.

Table 2. Comparison of patients with and without combined endpoint.

Parameters	Without Combined Endpoint ($n = 47$)	With Combined Endpoint ($n = 76$)	p-Value
		Clinical	
Age, years	55 (47–58)	55 (46–59)	0.7
Sex (male/female), n	42/5	61/15	$\chi^2 = 1.8; p = 0.2$
FC, NYHA (II/III/IV)	24/18/5	22/34/20	$\chi^2 = 7.6; p = 0.022$
Smoking status, n	28	41	$\chi^2 = 0.4; p = 0.53$
BMI, kg/m^2	26.3 (24; 33)	25.9 (22; 31)	0.44
Ischemic etiology, n	29	48	$\chi^2 = 0.06; p = 0.8$
LVEF Simpson, %	26 (20–29)	22 (16–27)	0.005
Epworth scale, points	5 (2–10)	6 (3–11)	0.7
CKD (eGFR < 60 mL/min/1.73 m^2), n	11	24	$\chi^2 = 1.2; p = 0.28$

Table 2. Cont.

Parameters	Without Combined Endpoint (n = 47)	With Combined Endpoint (n = 76)	p-Value
	Biomarkers *		
NT-proBNP, pg/mL (0–125)	619 (401–676)	2464 (928–4955)	0.001
sST-2, ng/mL (<35)	33 (31–35)	27 (24–34)	0.5
CRP, mg/mL (<5)	3 (1.8–7.7)	3.2 (1.7–5.9)	0.1
	Blood parameters *		
Uric acid, mcmol/L (210–420 male, 150–350 female)	510 (425–673)	480 (351–663)	0.21
eGFR (CKDEPI), mL/min/1.73 m^2	72 (59–82)	79 (51–84)	0.95
Total cholesterol, mmol/L (<5.0)	5.0 (3.7–5.8)	3.6 (3–5.8)	0.14
HDL, mmol/L (>1.0 male >1.2 female)	0.9 (0.8–1.1)	1.1 (0.6–1.6)	0.4
LDL, mmol/L (<3.0)	3.2 (2.5–3.9)	2.3 (2.1–3.4)	0.5
	PSG parameters		
AHI, episodes/h	26 (11–47)	12 (8–34)	0.9
OAI, episodes/h	0.6 (0–10)	0.7 (0.2–4)	0.1
CAI, episodes/h	3 (0.05–15)	0.6 (0–4)	0.4
MAI, episodes/h	7 (0–13)	0.7 (0–2.5)	0.4
HAI, episodes/h	11 (8–15)	10 (7–12)	0.088
ODI, episodes/h	29 (12–50)	15 (9–24)	0.3
SpO_2 Ave, %	93 (92–95)	94 (93–96)	0.4
SpO_2 Min, %	81 (77–88)	85 (79–87)	0.5
S_2, %	51 (44–56)	43 (31–56)	0.007
WASO, min	20 (9–76)	108 (38–143)	0.003
Mean duration of apnea, sec.	22 (20–28)	23 (19–28)	0.97
Max duration of apnea, sec.	47 (35–76)	49 (35–70)	0.7
	Cardiopulmonary exercise testing		
$VO_{2\,peak}$, mL/kg/min	18 (13–20)	15 (11–18)	0.003
VE/VCO_2 slope	34 (31–42)	41 (36–56)	0.004

AHI—apnea–hypopnea index, CAI—central apnea index, CKD-EPI—Chronic Kidney Disease Epidemiology Collaboration, CRP—C-reactive protein, eGFR—estimated glomerular filtration rate, FC—functional class, HAI—hypopnea index, HDL—high-density lipoproteins, LDL—low-density lipoproteins, LVEF—left ventricular ejection fraction, MAI—mixed apnea index, NT-proBNP—the N-terminal prohormone of brain natriuretic peptide, OAI—obstructive apnea index, ODI—oxygen desaturation index, S_2—duration of sleep stage 2, SpO_2 Ave and SpO_2 Min—average and minimum saturation O_2, sST2—soluble form of suppression of tumorigenicity-2, TST—total sleep time, VE/VCO_2 slope—the ventilator equivalent of CO_2, VO_2 peak—peak oxygen consumption, WASO—wake after sleep onset, sleep efficiency. *—normal values are indicated in brackets. Values are indicated as median (1st and 3rd quartiles).

Compared to the group without a combined endpoint, the group with adverse outcomes had higher NYHA classes, a lower LVEF, a higher NT-proBNP, a lower peak oxygen consumption, and a higher ventilator equivalent of CO_2. In patients with adverse events, AHI, SpO2, and ODI were comparable to patients without events. However, event patients had a significantly longer WASO time and shorter duration of S_2 (Table 2).

To investigate the predictive abilities of different parameters, a ROC curve analysis was constructed (Table 3 and Figures 1–3).

Table 3. ROC-curve analysis of clinical, laboratory and instrumental parameters.

Parameter	AUC	SE	AS	Asymptotic 95% CI	
				Lower Bound	Upper Bound
Age	0.498	0.054	0.976	0.393	0.604
BMI	0.458	0.055	0.443	0.351	0.565
NTproBNP	0.888	0.054	0.001	0.782	0.994
CRP	0.602	0.053	0.067	0.497	0.707
eGFR (CKDEPI)	0.485	0.054	0.789	0.380	0.591
VO_{2peak}	0.287	0.066	0.003	0.157	0.416
VO_2/HR	0.426	0.073	0.329	0.282	0.570
VE/VCO_2	0.709	0.073	0.004	0.566	0.852
LVEF	0.349	0.051	0.006	0.249	0.449
Sleep efficiency	0.447	0.059	0.373	0.331	0.562
AHI, episodes/h	0.488	0.058	0.835	0.375	0.602
TST	0.426	0.059	0.214	0.310	0.541
S_2	0.339	0.055	0.007	0.232	0.446
WASO	0.824	0.080	0.004	0.668	0.980
SpO_2Ave	0.550	0.057	0.379	0.439	0.661

AHI—apnea-hypopnea index, BMI—body mass index, CRP—C-reactive protein, CKD-EPI—Chronic Kidney Disease Epidemiology Collaboration, eGFR—estimated glomerular filtration rate, LVEF—left ventricular ejection fraction, NT-proBNP—the N-terminal prohormone of brain natriuretic peptide, S_2—duration of sleep stage 2, SpO_2Ave—average saturation O_2, TST—total sleep time, VO_2/HR (heart rate) oxygen pulse, VO_2 peak—peak oxygen consumption, VE/VCO_2 slope—the ventilator equivalent of CO_2. AS—asymptotic significance, AUC—area under curve, CI—confidence interval, SE—standard error.

We analyzed cut-offs of identified significant parameters that would better identify patients at high risk of adverse outcomes. A significantly higher risk of adverse events was observed in patients with LVEF ≤ 25.5%, NT-proBNP > 680 pg/mL, VO_{2peak} < 16 mL/kg/min, VE/VCO_2 slope ≥ 38.5, S_2 <44%, and WASO > 40 min.

The Kaplan–Meier analysis demonstrated that the combined endpoint significantly differs between LVEF categories, NTpro-BNP categories (Figure 4), VO_2peak categories, VE/VCO_2 slope categories (Figure 5), WASO categories, and S_2 categories (Figure 6).

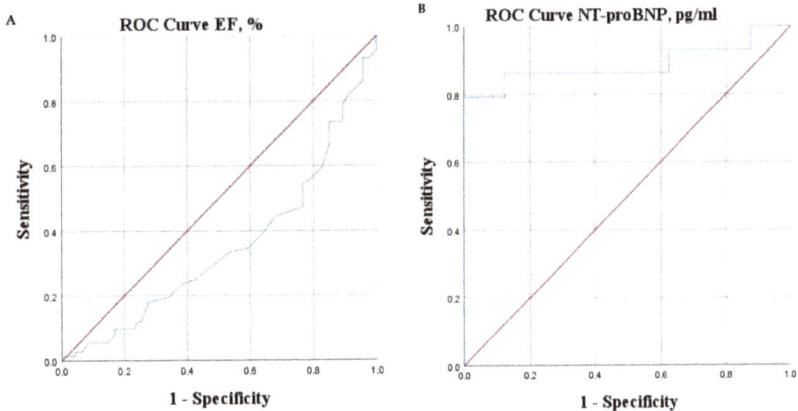

Figure 1. ROC curves of LVEF (**A**) and NT-pro-BNP (**B**).

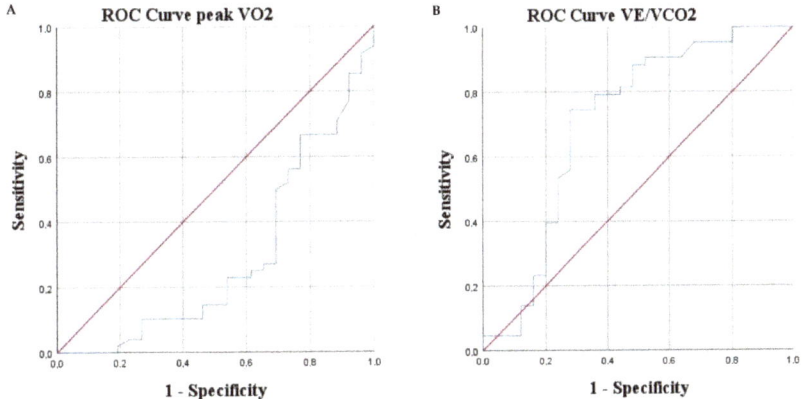

Figure 2. ROC curves of CPET parameters: VO_2peak (**A**), VE/VCO_2 (**B**).

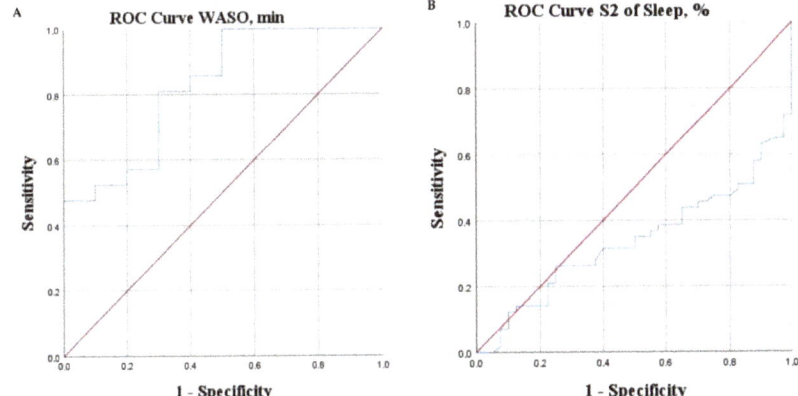

Figure 3. ROC curves of PSG parameters: WASO (**A**), S_2 (**B**).

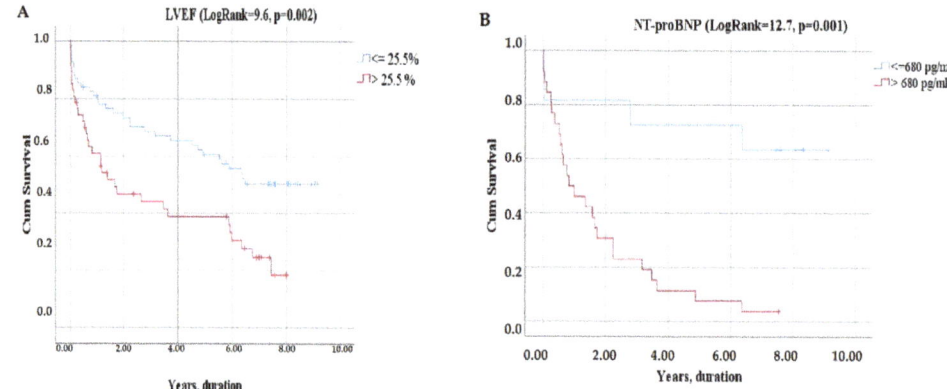

Figure 4. Kaplan–Meier curves of event-free survival according LVEF (**A**), NT-proBNP (**B**).

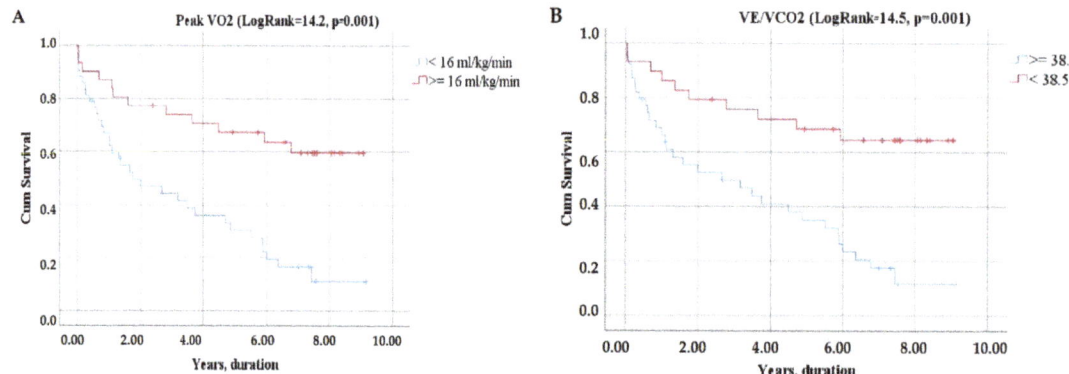

Figure 5. Kaplan–Meier curves of event-free survival according to CPET parameters: VO_2peak (**A**), VE/VCO_2 (**B**).

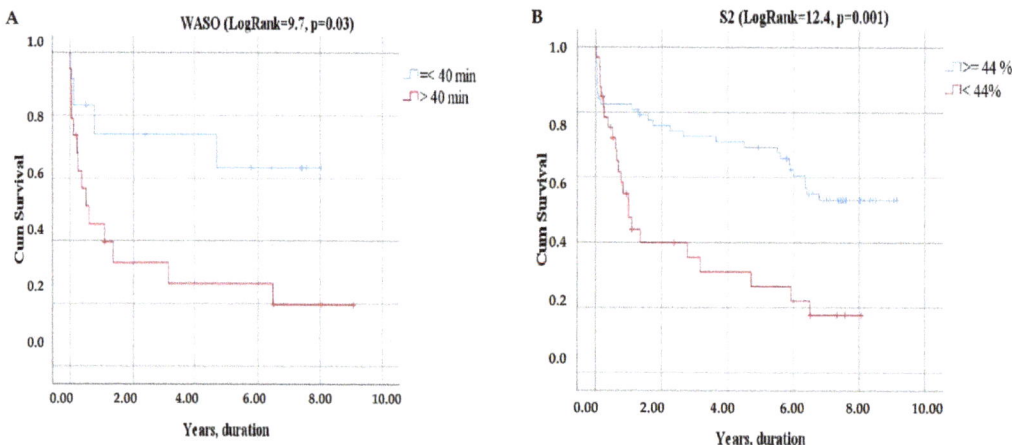

Figure 6. Kaplan–Meier curves of event-free survival according to PSG parameters: WASO (**A**), S_2 (**B**).

The proportion of patients surviving 8 years was significantly lower in patients with LVEF $\leq$ 25.50% compared to LVEF > 25.5%—0% vs. 19% (χ^2 = 9.6, log rank p = 0.002) (Figure 4A).

There was also an observed difference in survival between HF patients with NT-proBNP level > 680 pg/mL and those with an NT-proBNP level $\leq$ 680 pg/mL (χ^2 = 12.7, log rank p = 0.001): eight-year survival was 4% vs. 36%, respectively (Figure 4B).

Eight-year survival was 2% for those with VO$_2$peak < 16 mL/kg/min, 23% for those with VO$_2$peak $\geq$ 16 mL/kg/min, 3% for patients with VE/VCO$_2$ slope $\geq$ 38.5, and 24% for those below this cut-off (Figure 5).

The patients with WASO > 40 min and S$_2$ <44% had 8-year survival rates of 5% and 3% compared to 8% and 19% for those with WASO $\leq$40 min and S$_2$ $\geq$ 44%, respectively (Figure 6).

4. Discussion

According to the present study, patients with adverse events had a comparable AHI to those without an endpoint (p = 0.9). The limited role of AHI in HF is noted by many authors [10,11]. The severity of apnea, and most importantly its effect on outcomes, may be determined not only by AHI. This problem is discussed in the literature, and research is being conducted in this direction [12]. B. Gellen et al., demonstrated that the nocturnal desaturation is a marker of poor prognosis and helps identify high-risk patients. Moreover, severe nocturnal desaturation is associated with a poor prognosis, regardless of the existence of significant sleep apnea [13]. The authors described four different phenotypes depending on the presence of sleep apnea and minimal nocturnal oxygen saturation during sleep $\leq$ 88%.

Y. Huang et al., in a prospective cohort study, also demonstrated the prognostic role of nocturnal hypoxemia in patients with HF. A multivariate Cox regression analysis found that a saturation below 90% was independently associated with the outcome (hazard ratio [HR] 1.008, 95% confidence interval [CI] 1.001–1.016, p = 0.033), while no such association was found for AHI [11]. However, in the present study, the group with adverse events and the group without a combined endpoint had a comparable SpO$_{2ave}$ (p = 0.4), SpO$_{2min}$ (p = 0.5), ODI (p = 0.3), according to ROC analysis. AUC for SpO$_2$ was 0.55 (95%CI 0.439–0.661, p = 0.057). This can be explained by different designs and methods. In their study, Huang Y. et al., included patients with acute decompensated HF and used a portable screening device (class 4 equipment with certain limitations) rather than full PSG, which is explained by the clinical status of patients. In our study, patients showed no evidence of fluid overload and/or hypoperfusion at the time of PSG, in contrast to Huang's study. Such symptoms are associated with severe congestion in the lungs and hypoxia; therefore, in our opinion, it is difficult to identify the contribution of apnea to the development of hypoxia in patients with acute decompensation. Moreover, as previously stated, conducting a full PSG allowed us to obtain more data and include more variables in the analytical matrix.

Our results demonstrate that assessing the prognostic role of polysomnography indicators is a multicomponent problem, and a heterogeneous cohort of patients with heart failure with previous decompensation may have different PSG predictors of poor prognosis: WASO and duration of S$_2$. The current study also found other laboratory and instrumental parameters (NT-proBNP, VO$_2$peak, VE/VCO$_2$ slope) that were independent risk factors for a combined endpoint.

B. Yan et al., in a community-based cohort study (n = 3810), found that sleep efficiency and wake after sleep onset were predictors of major adverse cardiovascular events. Wake after sleep onset >78minutes was associated with primary (HR, 1.436; 95% CI, 1.066–1.934; p = 0.017) and secondary composite cardiovascular outcomes (HR, 1.374; 95% CI, 1.103–1.712; p = 0.005), as well as cardiovascular mortality (HR, 2.240; 95% CI, 1.377–3.642; p = 0.001) [14]. We also established the significant prognostic role of WASO, but with another cut-off level of >40 min, due to examination of a completely different cohort of patients. On the one hand, such an association can be explained by the presence of severe symptoms of HF in patients at night; on the other hand, long WASO may contribute to the progression of HF due to the activation of the sympathetic–adrenal system and other pathogenetic factors (endothelial damage and dysfunction, progression of atherosclerosis, etc.) [15].

The present study has the following limitations: first of all, a relatively small sample size can reduce the generalizability of the predictive value of PSG and other parameters. The studied cohort is heterogeneous in terms of LVEF, functional classes, and the etiology of HF. However, we recruited patients who were stabilized after previous decompensation of HF and aimed to identify the role of PSG indicators in prognosis.

Thus, according to our results, we can conclude that WASO > 40 min and S_2 <44% were independent predictors of a combined endpoint in patients with previous decompensation of HF. These PSG parameters may be used for estimation prognosis as well as NT-proBNP, LVEF, VE/VCO$_2$ slope, and VO$_{2peak}$.

Author Contributions: Conceptualization, E.M. and Y.S. (Yurii Sviryaev); methodology, E.M., L.K., M.B. and A.B.; software, L.K. and Y.S. (Yurii Sviryaev); validation, E.M., Y.S. (Yurii Sviryaev) and L.K.; formal analysis, E.M., A.S. and Y.S. (Yurii Sviryaev); investigation, E.M., L.K., A.S., Y.S. (Yulia Sazonova), A.B., M.B., M.S. and A.K.; resources, Y.S. (Yurii Sviryaev), A.B., Y.S. (Yulia Sazonova) and M.S.; data curation, E.M., L.K., A.S., Y.S. (Yulia Sazonova), M.B., A.B., M.S., Y.S. (Yurii Sviryaev) and A.K.; writing—original draft preparation, E.M. and L.K.; writing—review and editing, E.M., L.K., M.S. and M.B.; visualization, E.M. and Y.S. (Yurii Sviryaev); supervision, E.M. and Y.S. (Yurii Sviryaev); project administration, A.S., M.S., A.K. and Y.S. (Yulia Sazonova). All authors have read and agreed to the published version of the manuscript.

Funding: This work was financially supported by the Ministry of Science and Higher Education of the Russian Federation (Agreement No. 075-15-2022-301).

Institutional Review Board Statement: The study was conducted in accordance with the Declaration of Helsinki, and approved by the Ethics Committee of Almazov National Medical Research Centre (protocol code 14623/2012, date of approval 3 February 2012).

Informed Consent Statement: Informed consent was obtained from all subjects involved in the study.

Data Availability Statement: Data is contained within the article.

Acknowledgments: Special thanks to Maria Yu. Sitnikova, Petr A. Fedotov for their leadership in heart failure healthcare at Almazov National Medical Research Centre and support in manuscript preparation.

Conflicts of Interest: The authors declare no conflict of interest.

References

1. Parati, G.; Lombardi, C.; Castagna, F.; Mattaliano, P.; Filardi, P.P.; Agostoni, P. and Italian Society of Cardiology Working Group on Heart Failure: Heart failure and sleep disorders. *Nat. Rev. Cardiol.* **2016**, *13*, 389–403. [CrossRef] [PubMed]
2. Lyngkaran, P.; Liew, D.; Neil, C.; Driscoll, A.; Hare, D.L. Moving from Heart Failure Guidelines to Clinical Practice: Gaps Contributing to Readmissions in Patients with Multiple Comorbidities and Older Age. *Clin. Med. Insights: Cardiol.* **2018**, *12*, 1179546818809358. [CrossRef]
3. Khayat, R.; Jarjoura, D.; Porter, K.; Sow, A.; Wannemacher, J.; Dohar, R.; Pleister, A.; Abraham, W.T. Sleep disordered breathing and post-discharge mortality in patients with acute heart failure. *Eur. Heart J.* **2015**, *36*, 1463–1469. [CrossRef] [PubMed]
4. Bitter, T.; Westerheide, N.; Prinz, C.; Hossain, M.S.; Vogt, J.; Langer, C.; Horstkotte, D.; Oldenburg, O. Cheyne-Stokes respiration and obstructive sleep apnoea are independent risk factors for malignant ventricular arrhythmias requiring appropriate cardioverter-defibrillator therapies in patients with congestive heart failure. *Eur. Heart J.* **2011**, *32*, 61–74. [CrossRef] [PubMed]
5. Gottlieb, D.J.; Yenokyan, G.; Newman, A.B.; O'Connor, G.T.; Punjabi, N.M.; Quan, S.F.; Redline, S.; Resnick, H.E.; Tong, E.K.; Diener-West, M.; et al. Prospective study of obstructive sleep apnea and incident coronary heart disease and heart failure: The sleep heart health study. *Circulation* **2010**, *122*, 352–360. [CrossRef] [PubMed]
6. Grimm, W.; Sosnovskaya, A.; Timmesfeld, N.; Hildebrandt, O.; Koehler, U. Prognostic impact of central sleep apnea in patients with heart failure. *J. Card. Fail.* **2015**, *21*, 126–133. [CrossRef] [PubMed]
7. American Academy of Sleep Medicine Task Force. Sleep-related breathing disorders in adults: Recommendations for syndrome definition and measurement technique in clinical research. The report of an American Academy of Sleep Medicine Task Force. *Sleep* **1999**, *22*, 667–689. [CrossRef]

8. Lang, R.M.; Badano, L.P.; Mor-Avi, V.; Afilalo, J.; Armstrong, A.; Ernande, L.; Flachskampf, F.A.; Foster, E.; Goldstein, S.A.; Kuznetsova, T.; et al. Recommendations for cardiac chamber quantification by echocardiography in adults: An update from the American Society of Echocardiography and the European Association of Cardiovascular Imaging. *Eur. Heart J. Cardiovasc. Imaging* **2015**, *16*, 233–270. [CrossRef] [PubMed]
9. Galderisi, M.; Cosyns, B.; Edvardsen, T.; Cardim, N.; Delgado, V.; Di Salvo, G.; Donal, E.; Sade, L.E.; Ernande, L.; Garbi, M.; et al. 2016–2018 EACVI Scientific Documents Committee. Standardization of adult transthoracic echocardiography reporting in agreement with recent chamber quantification, diastolic function, and heart valve disease recommendations: An expert consensus document of the European Association of Cardiovascular Imaging. *Eur. Heart J. Cardiovasc. Imaging* **2017**, *18*, 1301–1310. [CrossRef] [PubMed]
10. Efken, C.; Bitter, T.; Prib, N.; Horstkotte, D.; Oldenburg, O. Obstructive sleep apnoea: Longer respiratory event lengths in patients with heart failure. *Eur. Respir. J.* **2013**, *41*, 1340–1346. [CrossRef] [PubMed]
11. Huang, Y.; Wang, Y.; Huang, Y.; Zhai, M.; Zhou, Q.; Zhao, X.; Tian, P.; Ji, S.; Zhang, C.; Zhang, J. Prognostic value of sleep apnea and nocturnal hypoxemia in patients with decompensated heart failure. *Clin. Cardiol.* **2020**, *43*, 329–337. [CrossRef]
12. Tam, S.; Woodson, B.T.; Rotenberg, B. Outcome measurements in obstructive sleep apnea: Beyond the apnea-hypopnea index. *Laryngoscope* **2014**, *124*, 337–343. [CrossRef]
13. Gellen, B.; Canouï-Poitrine, F.; Boyer, L.; Drouot, X.; Le Thuaut, A.; Bodez, D.; Covali-Noroc, A.; D'Ortho, M.P.; Guendouz, S.; Rappeneau, S.; et al. Apnea-hypopnea and desaturations in heart failure with reduced ejection fraction: Are we aiming at the right target? *Int. J. Cardiol.* **2016**, *203*, 1022–1028. [CrossRef]
14. Yan, B.; Yang, J.; Zhao, B.; Fan, Y.; Wang, W.; Ma, X. Objective Sleep Efficiency Predicts Cardiovascular Disease in a Community Population: The Sleep Heart Health Study. *J. Am. Heart Assoc.* **2021**, *10*, e016201. [CrossRef]
15. Von Kanel, R.; Loredo, J.S.; Ancoli-Israel, S.; Mills, P.J.; Natarajan, L.; Dimsdale, J.E. Association between polysomnographic measures of disrupted sleep and prothrombotic factors. *Chest* **2007**, *131*, 733–739. [CrossRef] [PubMed]

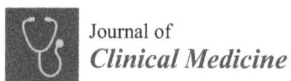

Review

The Role of Novel Cardiac Imaging for Contemporary Management of Heart Failure

Frank A. Flachskampf [1,*] and Tomasz Baron [1,2]

1. Department of Medical Sciences, Cardiology and Clinical Physiology, Uppsala University Hospital, Uppsala University, 751 85 Uppsala, Sweden
2. Uppsala Clinical Research Center, Uppsala University, 752 36 Uppsala, Sweden
* Correspondence: frank.flachskampf@medsci.uu.se

Abstract: Heart failure is becoming the central problem in cardiology. Its recognition, differential diagnosis, and the monitoring of therapy are intimately coupled with cardiac imaging. Cardiac imaging has witnessed an explosive growth and differentiation, with echocardiography continuing as the first diagnostic step; the echocardiographic exam itself has become considerably more complex than in the last century, with the assessment of diastolic left ventricular function and strain imaging contributing important information, especially in heart failure. Very often, however, echocardiography can only describe the fact of functional impairment and morphologic remodeling, whereas further clarification of the underlying disease, such as cardiomyopathy, myocarditis, storage diseases, sarcoidosis, and others, remains elusive. Here, cardiovascular magnetic resonance and perfusion imaging should be used judiciously to arrive as often as possible at a clear diagnosis which ideally enables specific therapy.

Keywords: heart failure; cardiac imaging; echocardiography; cardiac magnetic resonance; computed tomography; positron emission tomography

Citation: Flachskampf, F.A.; Baron, T. The Role of Novel Cardiac Imaging for Contemporary Management of Heart Failure. *J. Clin. Med.* **2022**, *11*, 6201. https://doi.org/10.3390/jcm11206201

Academic Editors: Mario J. Garcia and Fatih Yalcin

Received: 8 September 2022
Accepted: 16 October 2022
Published: 20 October 2022

Publisher's Note: MDPI stays neutral with regard to jurisdictional claims in published maps and institutional affiliations.

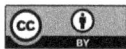

Copyright: © 2022 by the authors. Licensee MDPI, Basel, Switzerland. This article is an open access article distributed under the terms and conditions of the Creative Commons Attribution (CC BY) license (https://creativecommons.org/licenses/by/4.0/).

1. Introduction

Heart failure, typically and somewhat vaguely defined as a condition in which the heart is unable to pump enough blood to meet the body's needs, has grown into one of the most important cardiovascular health challenges, in part due to an ageing population, in part due to the improved treatment of conditions formerly leading to earlier death, such as myocardial infarction, which now are more likely to being survived, but nevertheless may lead to later heart failure. In Sweden, about 2% of the population are affected by clinically manifested heart failure [1].

"Heart failure" comprises a multitude of etiologies and pathophysiologies, and is in itself a rather broad concept defined by a constellation of clinical symptoms and signs. Therefore, to provide management and therapy tailored to individual etiology, as specific a diagnosis as possible is necessary. In the majority of cases, cardiac imaging is necessary—and often sufficient—to arrive at such specific diagnoses, complemented by laboratory chemistry and invasive diagnostics, where necessary. Cardiac imaging in heart failure has evolved over roughly the last 50 years from chest X-ray, until very recently a nearly always-obtained test, to the impressive armamentarium available—in spite of some restrictions—today. In this article, we will review the capabilities of current cardiac imaging according to clinical questions in the context of heart failure.

2. Is It Heart Failure?

Remarkably, the basic diagnosis of heart failure remains largely a clinical one based on history, physical examination, and natriuretic peptides. Although, for example, pulmonary congestion is very well detectable by radiology or lung ultrasound, milder forms of heart failure are difficult to pin down with confidence without suggestive symptoms and signs. In this context, natriuretic peptides have largely superseded the use of the chest X-ray to screen for heart failure, although they are multifactorial, sex- and body-mass-dependent, may increase in response to heart failure medication (e.g., beta blockers), have a large scatter, and have limited accuracy in milder forms of heart failure [2].

3. Valvular Heart Disease

Severe—and sometimes moderate—primary valvular heart disease is an important cause or contributor to heart failure. Since this etiology is frequently and well described in the current literature, this review does not include a detailed discussion of valvular heart disease.

4. Left and Right Ventricular Function

Left ventricular (LV) "function" is a fuzzy term, but overwhelmingly important in cardiologists' thinking. Systolic LV function is mostly equated with ejection fraction (EF) or global longitudinal strain (GLS), although an argument could be made for using stroke volume or stroke work instead. Stroke volume, and its product with heart rate, cardiac output, is "what the body sees" of the ventricles' performance, and is typically reduced in heart failure with reduced EF, but also in heart failure with preserved EF, thus offering a more uniform physiologic correlate of the clinical syndrome of heart failure. As a clinical illustration, take the scenarios of manifested cardiac amyloidosis or of papillary muscle rupture, both leading to normal or even high ejection fraction, together with critically reduced stroke volume. This can be further refined by correcting for afterload, e.g., by multiplying stroke volume by mean arterial blood pressure to yield stroke work.

"Diastolic function", an even less clear term, describes the complex variations in LV diastolic pressure–volume relationships, and is typically assessed by indirect echocardiographic signs, which have modest accuracy at best [3,4].

Heart failure diagnosis is now tightly related to the determination of left ventricular ejection fraction (EF) by virtue of the current stratification of heart failure into three subgroups of heart failure according to their EF, heart failure with reduced EF (HFrEF), heart failure with mildly reduced EF (HFmrEF), and heart failure with preserved EF (HFpEF) [2].

Ejection fraction is routinely measured by 2D echocardiography, with acceptable accuracy compared to the gold standard CMR. LV volumes (both end-diastolic and end-systolic), however, are regularly and substantially underestimated by 2D echocardiography. This can be partly overcome by 3D echocardiography and/or left heart contrast use. 3D echocardiography also compensates for irregularities in ventricular shape, such as in aneurysms, but depends on good image quality.

Additionally, the newer speckle tracking-based deformation parameter, global longitudinal shortening (GLS), serves mainly as a sort of canary in the mine in the presence of borderline or slightly reduced EF; for example, in valvular heart disease or cardiotoxicity of cancer therapy, where GLS decreases earlier and by a higher proportion than EF in the early stages and, therefore, regularly pre-dates later EF reductions [5]. In direct comparison, the prognostic value of GLS regularly outperforms EF [6] in patients with heart failure, probably because of better discrimination at the lower limits of normalcy. The reasons for this superiority of GLS over EF are not entirely clear. Higher sensitivity of longitudinal LV function for subtle functional changes seems to be essential, since longitudinal function is more directly measured by GLS than by EF.

The assessment of diastolic function has recently been improved, with added prognostic value, by adding left atrial (LA) strain to the diagnostic algorithm ([7,8]; Figures 1 and 2). Other important developments in the non-invasive diagnosis of diastolic LV dysfunction are the use of provocative maneuvers such as physical exercise or volume challenge [9–11]. Such maneuvers aim to unmask diastolic dysfunction which may not be evident at rest by increasing cardiac workload. Under provocation by exercise or volume, LV stiffness increases and leads to measurable changes in indirect parameters such as E/e' or right ventricular systolic pressure. Other experimental techniques assess the twisting and untwisting motion of the LV around its long axis, which are important for both systolic (twist) and diastolic (untwist) LV function; this can be accomplished by speckle-tracking echocardiography or CMR [12]. Finally, shear wave imaging, which harnesses the information on tissue stiffness from the velocity of pressure waves in the myocardium, may be useful if it can be standardized and technically integrated in ultrasound machines ([13,14]; Figure 3).

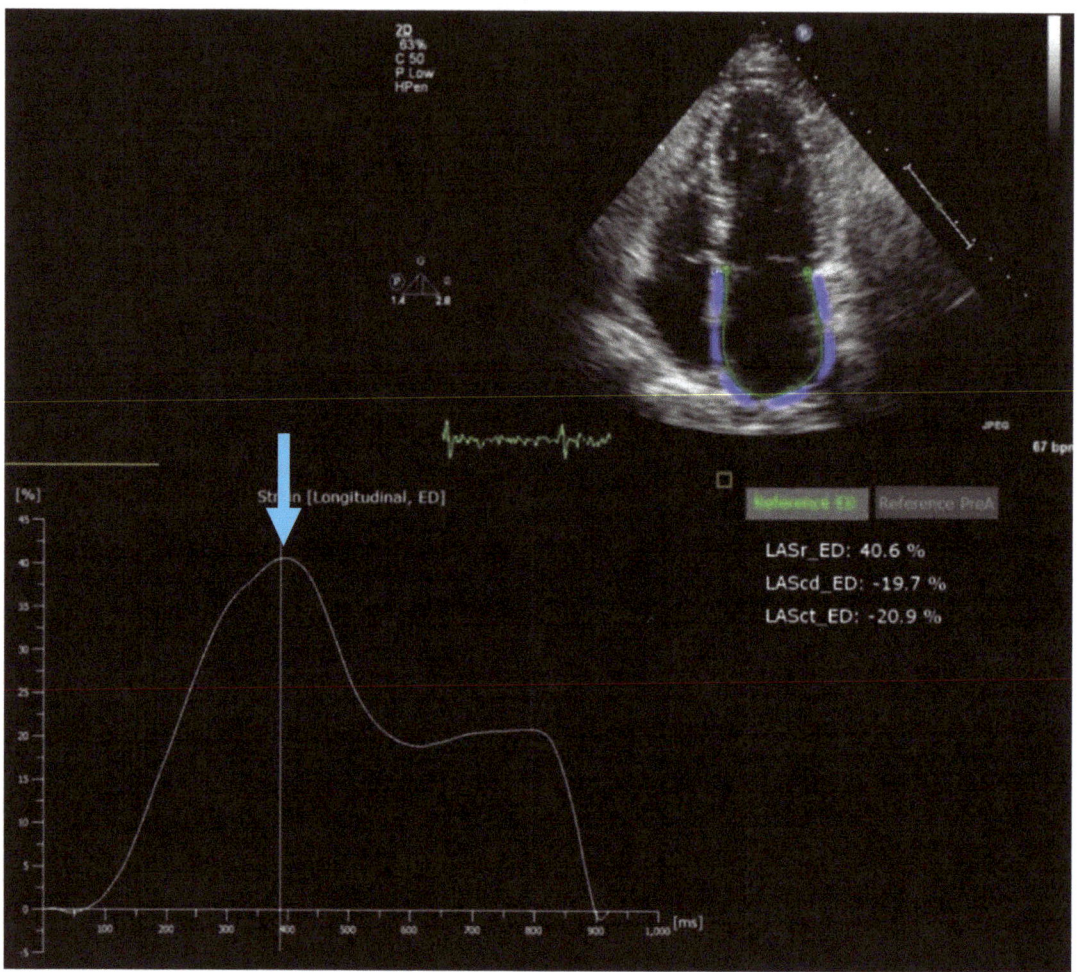

Figure 1. Left atrial strain by speckle tracking echocardiography. Upper panel: echocardiographic image (apical four-chamber view) showing the left ventricle (LV) and left atrium (LA) with blue coded region of interest for LA strain tracking. Lower panel: LA strain trace along with ECG. Reservoir strain (41%) is indicated by the blue arrow.

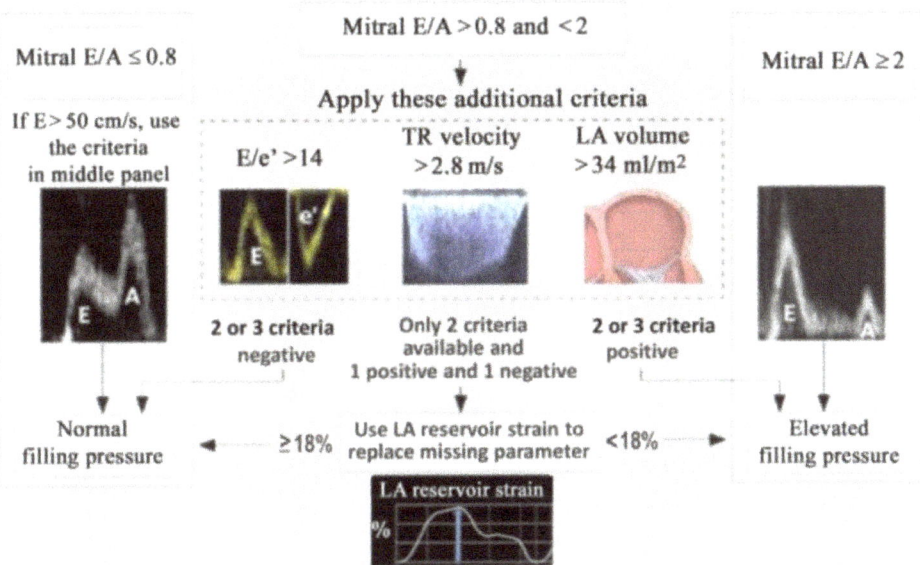

Figure 2. Current algorithm of the European Association of Cardiovascular Imaging for echocardiographic assessment of left ventricular filling pressure in patients with suspected heart failure with preserved ejection fraction. Note that this algorithm integrates left atrial reservoir strain, with a cut-off of 18%, as a reserve parameter if one of the classic parameters, LA volume, E/e', or systolic pulmonary arterial pressure, cannot be obtained with confidence. Reproduced, with permission, from [8].

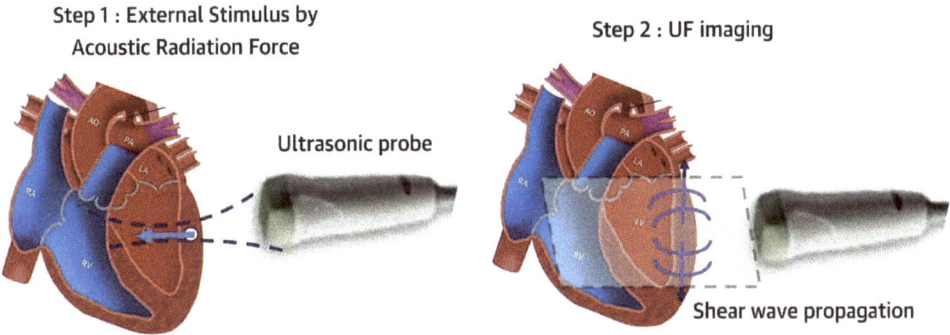

Figure 3. Schematic drawing of externally stimulated shear wave imaging. The shear wave is initiated by an external stimulus, and then visualized by very-high-framerate imaging. This allows imaging the propagation of the shear wave, and to obtain shear wave speed. From shear wave speed, under simplifying assumptions, the stiffness of a tissue can be calculated. UF ultrafast. Adapted with permission from [14].

An important, but underappreciated, area of echocardiographic imaging is patients with impaired LV function with left bundle branch block who are candidates for cardiac resynchronization therapy. Although past trials have had mixed results for the predictability of CRT success from baseline echocardiographic parameters, several visual features ("mechanical abnormalities") have been described which imply an increased likelihood for a benefit from CRT: (1) the septal flash, (2) "apical rocking", etc. [15].

Right ventricular (RV) function is more difficult to quantify, given the more limited visualization by echo, the complex RV morphology with separate inflow and outflow tract, and the stronger impact of preload and afterload on all RV functional parameters. The classic echo parameters, such as tricuspid annular plane systolic excursion (TAPSE) and fractional area change, have been complemented by RV strain, both in its "global" (six segments) or free wall strain (three segments) form, but the obtained strain only reflects myocardial shortening of the RV seen in the apical four-chamber view, i.e., the inflow tract of the RV. Even more limited, and essentially a close relative of TAPSE, is the basal RV free wall's systolic peak velocity S'. Three-dimensional echocardiography, although often impractical due to image quality, can provide the EF of the entire RV, which is generally accepted as the best parameter of RV function. RVEF can be obtained with greater accuracy and more reliable absolute RV volumes by CMR and CT. Therefore, if RV performance needs to be assessed and monitored with high precision, e.g., in postoperative Fallot tetralogy patients with substantial pulmonary regurgitation, CMR is now the preferred modality. It should be remembered, however, that all of the cited global left or right ventricular functional parameters are clearly dependent on preload and afterload, and have substantial test–retest variability [16,17]. Parameters which include or correct for afterload, such as stroke work or cardiac power output [18,19], or true myocardial external efficiency based on myocardial oxygen uptake [20] obtained by positron emission tomography (PET) have not reached clinical implementation, in spite of some encouraging data in the literature. Very recently, the myocardial work "index" derived from pressure-strain loops of the left ventricle, which can be obtained non-invasively by the extrapolation of cuff blood pressure recordings, has been proposed as a parameter incorporating blood pressure as a measure of afterload. This approach, however, was originally developed to detect regional differences in mechanical work, such as those occurring in left bundle branch block. It does not take into account absolute ventricular volumes, and, therefore, is best suited for intra-individual comparisons, e.g., before and after cardiac resynchronization, where "wasted work" of the septum in left bundle branch block conditions can be measured, and the benefit from resynchronization quantified regionally [21–25]. For the performance of the right ventricle, recently, the ratio of TAPSE to systolic pulmonary arterial pressure (SPAP), sometimes described as an index of ventriculo-arterial loading, has been proposed [26]. This index has shown prognostic value, e.g., in patients with heart failure [26], medically treated tricuspid regurgitation [27], and in patients undergoing mitral edge-to-edge repair for functional mitral regurgitation [28], but not in other studies, e.g., in the context of transcatheter tricuspid valve repair [29].

5. Cardiac Imaging for Monitoring Heart Failure

In some clinical situations, it is desirable to not only monitor patients' symptoms (and natriuretic peptides) under heart failure therapy, but also to quantify objectively functional improvements and reverse remodeling of the heart. An example of this is the recommendation to defer implantation of a prophylactic implantable cardioverter/defibrillator in patients with newly diagnosed HFrEF with EF $\leq$ 35% for at least 3 months to allow for recovery of LV function under "optimal medical therapy". It should be pointed out that though therapy with angiotensin-converting enzyme inhibitors, beta blockers, and sacubitril/valsartan leads to a well-documented improvement in ejection fraction, this effect seems to be absent or minor in SGLT2 inhibitors [30,31].

6. Structure of the Myocardium

Though echocardiography delineates well the border between blood and tissue, and furnishes fundamental, if not very precise, information about linear dimensions and volumes of chambers, the characterization of the chamber walls themselves is very limited. In a very approximative way, LV mass is assessed using linear dimensions at the base of the LV, and LV hypertrophy is, thus, diagnosed clinically. Note, however, that this is essentially a misnomer, since we are simply converting wall volume into mass by multiplying cm^3 (or mL) by 1.04 g/mL to arrive at grams. This volume-derived mass may be hypertrophied myocytes, as in hypertension or aortic stenosis, but it may also be due to an increase in extracellular space, as in cardiac amyloidosis, myocardial edema, diffuse or localized ("replacement") fibrosis, intracellular glycosphingolipids in Fabry disease [32], and others. Echocardiography may provide clues about specific diseases; for example, in cardiac amyloidosis, it has been observed that apical LV segments tend to have preserved longitudinal strain, whereas mid and basal segments display reduced strain ("apical sparing"; [33]). However, this sign lacks specificity in hypertrophied ventricles, and, in amyloidosis, becomes positive mainly in advanced disease. In some cases, as in aortic stenosis, we know that, besides true myocyte hypertrophy, 10–15% of patients also have cardiac amyloidosis [34], and, thus, these patients have both a myocardial and extracellular increase in mass. This blind spot for echocardiography can be removed to an extent by CMR and perfusion imaging.

"Virtual histology" by CMR is based on two principles [35]:

1. Early and late tissue enhancement after contrast (gadolinium) application allows separation of intact myocardium from extracellular space, since intact myocardiocytes do not allow the intracellular accumulation of gadolinium. Thus, late gadolinium enhancement can detect myocardial scars as locally increased extracellular volume, such as infarcts, post-myocarditis damage, sarcoidosis, and other localized increases of extracellular volume (Figure 4). This technique relies on relative contrast intensity differences between myocardial regions, as in a myocardial infarction, but does not work in the presence of diffuse alterations of extracellular space. Though all of the cited etiologies result in the formation of localized increases of extracellular volume, often the "gestalt" of such a region of late contrast enhancement suggests a specific etiology. For example, subendocardial or transmural late enhancement following the "wavefront phenomenon" of myocardial ischemia in a coronary perfusion territory is strongly suggestive of post-infarct scar, and mid-wall late enhancement, especially in the lateral wall, suggests post-myocarditis damage. Note that similar principles enable contrast-enhanced CT to diagnose localized increases in extracellular space [36] in a similar manner to CMR, although the achieved contrast between normal and diseased regions is weaker than with CMR techniques.

2. Pixel-wise maps of the magnetic relaxation parameters T1, T2, and T2*, called "parametric imaging", allow a limited characterization of underlying tissue ([37]; Figure 5). Additionally, by pre- and post-contrast registration of T1 in the myocardium and blood pool, a direct relative measure of extracellular volume (in percent) for each pixel can be calculated. For example, hemochromatosis leads to shortening and amyloidosis leads to lengthening of T1 relaxation times, which sets these pathologies apart from others. Myocardial edema leads to lengthening of T1 and T2 times and the expansion of extracellular volume, which in themselves are non-specific, but may aid in the diagnosis of, e.g., myocarditis, depending on clinical circumstances. Notably, increased extracellular space may be indicative of diffuse fibrosis but also, e.g., tissue edema. Hence, although, for example, an increased T1 value does correlate modestly with myocardial fibrosis and may, therefore, support the diagnosis of diastolic dysfunction and HFpEF, the relaxation parameters are multifactorial and should not be mistaken for true histology.

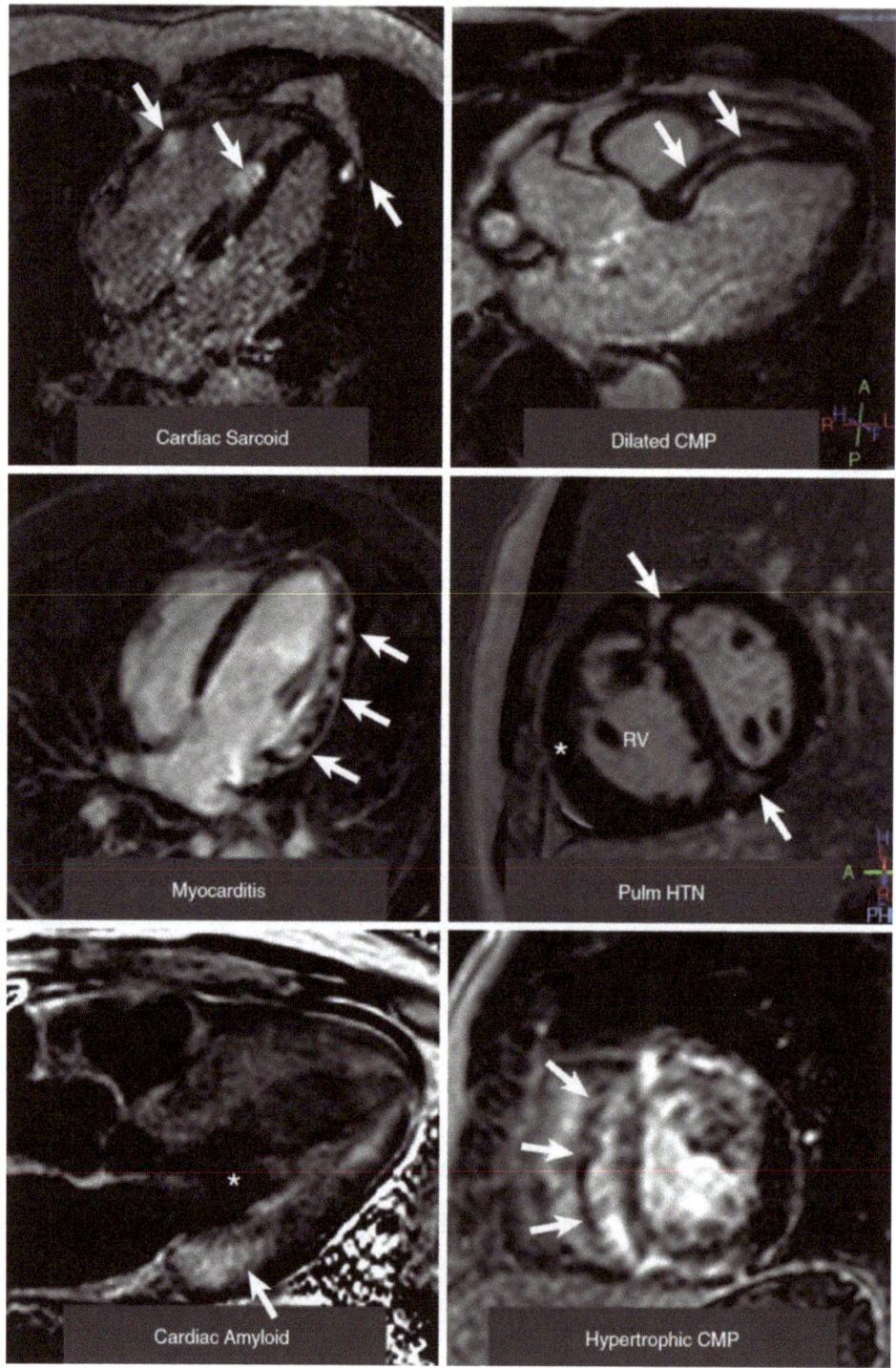

Figure 4. CMR images with late gadolinium enhancement (LGE) in non-ischemic cardiomyopathies. Top left: cardiac sarcoidosis, with patchy distribution of LGE (arrows) in lateral wall and septum. Top right:

septal mid-wall "stripe" pattern of LGE (arrows) in dilated cardiomyopathy. Middle left: patchy epicardial and mid-wall LGE (arrows) in the lateral wall in myocarditis. Middle right: midventricular short-axis view in a patient with pulmonary hypertension, right ventricular dilatation, and hypertrophy (star). Note LGE (arrows) at the right ventricular insertion points. Bottom left: cardiac amyloid. The LV blood pool is nulled (star) and there is subtle circumferential subendocardial LGE throughout the LV, most pronounced at the base (arrow). Bottom right: midventricular short-axis view of patient with hypertrophic cardiomyopathy and septal hypertrophy showing extensive mid-wall LGE (arrows). Reproduced, with permission, from [38].

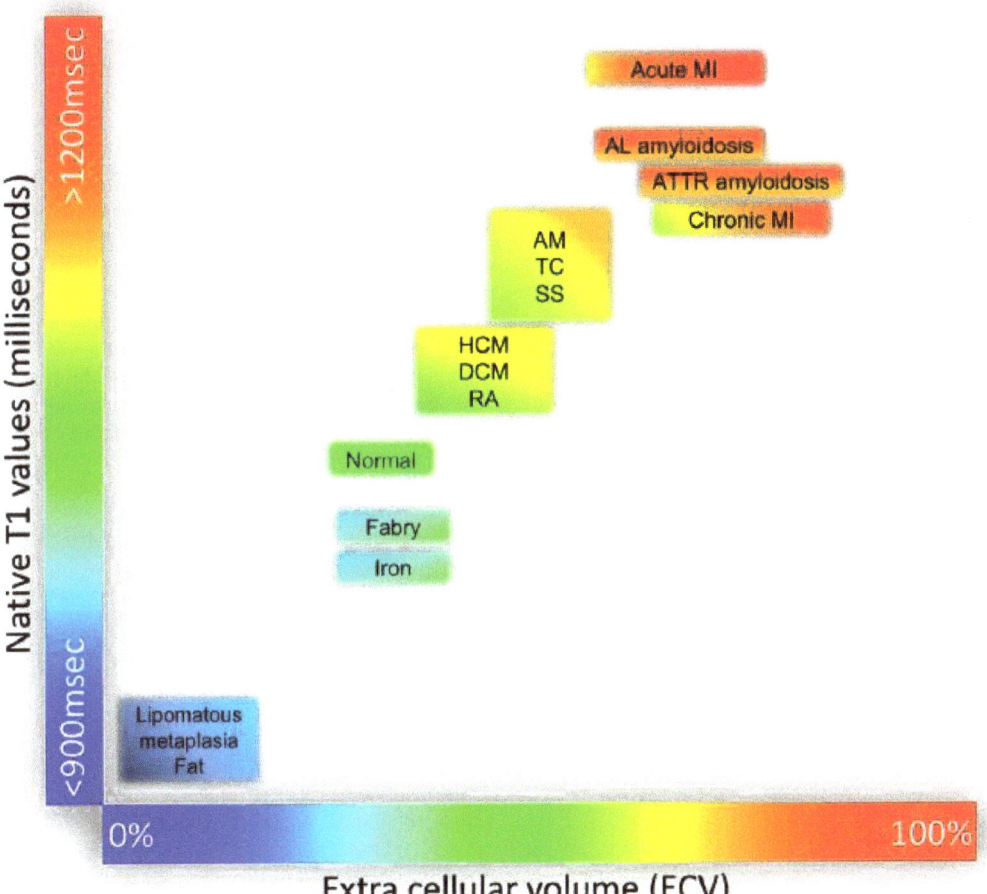

Figure 5. Tissue characterization using native T1 and extracellular volume fraction (ECV). For the purpose of comparability, only studies using 1.5 T scanners were considered in this figure. AM, acute myocarditis; DCM, dilated cardiomyopathy; HCM, hypertrophic cardiomyopathy; MI, myocardial infarction; RA, rheumatoid arthritis; TC, takotsubo cardiomyopathy; SS, systemic sclerosis. Reproduced according to the Creative Commons CC BY license from [39].

GLS by echocardiography or CMR has been shown to correlate with diffuse myocardial fibrosis, both for the left ventricle and for the left atrium [40,41], but the correlation is modest at best and is difficult to apply for individual clinical decisions. Similarly, clear signs of diastolic dysfunction, such as short E wave deceleration, high E/e' ratio, low left atrial strain, or increased systolic right ventricular pressure, are suggestive of increased diastolic LV pressures, which, in turn, are indicative of myocardial fibrosis, if other causes can be excluded. It should be clear, though, that CMR relaxation times or echocardiographic GLS are not specific histologic markers, and are, at best, modestly related to histological fibrosis.

7. Myocardial Perfusion

Coronary artery disease (CAD) is an important cause of heart failure, and the classic way to non-invasively diagnose CAD is diagnosing inducible ischemia. This is traditionally performed either by looking at LV wall motion abnormalities during physical or pharmacological stress by echocardiography [42], or, less frequently, by gated single-photon emission tomography (SPECT), or CMR cine-loops. Left heart echo contrast application improves the diagnostic accuracy of stress echocardiography, and should be strongly considered even in patients with acceptable image quality at rest [43]. The injection of contrast, besides opacification of the chambers, leads to myocardial opacification, and this can be used to assess myocardial perfusion. The technique is highly dependent on experienced operators, however, since the destruction of microbubbles by the ultrasound itself may mimic hypoperfusion. Several other refinements have been proposed, most importantly the recording of coronary flow velocity in the mid-left anterior descending coronary artery, coupled with a vasodilator stress (adenosine or dipyridamole) to determine coronary flow velocity reserve. Again, a learning curve exists, and the method has not found widespread acceptance.

Alternatively, perfusion can be directly visualized by nuclear imaging (SPECT or PET) or contrast CMR. Using specialized tracers, PET allows to obtain estimates of absolute regional perfusion (in mL blood per second and gram myocardium), and, thus, is able to assess perfusion at the myocardial level, enabling the evaluation of the whole cardiac vasculature. Further, contrast CMR [44] has been shown not only to be a highly accurate diagnostic method to diagnose ischemia, but also to provide strong prognostic data, and reduce the number of unnecessary invasive coronary angiographies in patients with stable chest pain [45]. Moreover, recently, quantitative myocardial blood flow mapping using CMR has also been introduced, offering the ability to separate epicardial multivessel disease from microvascular disease besides prognostic stratification [46,47].

A specific strength of PET is the possibility to characterize regional perfusion and metabolism using different tracers, enabling the detection of a myocardium which is metabolically active, but underperfused and non-functional, the classic hallmark of a viable myocardium. Although the clinical utility of diagnosing myocardial viability has been questioned due to lack of data showing prognostic benefit, most prominently in the STICH trial [48], there is ongoing clinical interest [49] in this scenario.

8. Other Nuclear Imaging

Nuclear imaging with non-perfusion tracers plays an important role in the diagnosis of several less frequent diseases causing heart failure. One of them, which is now treatable, is cardiac amyloidosis. ^{99m}Tc-3,3-diphosphono-1,2-propanodicarboxylic acid (DPD)-SPECT (or planar imaging), originally introduced as a "bone scan" for bone imaging, especially bone metastases, is an excellent tool for diagnosing ATTR amyloidosis. However, other forms of amyloidosis, especially AL amyloidosis, are not well detected by DPD imaging, and need blood or urine chemistry or specialized PET tracers [50] for diagnosis (Figure 6). Sarcoidosis, a rare but treatable cause of heart failure, is also well detected by PET, which has higher specificity than CMR for this disease.

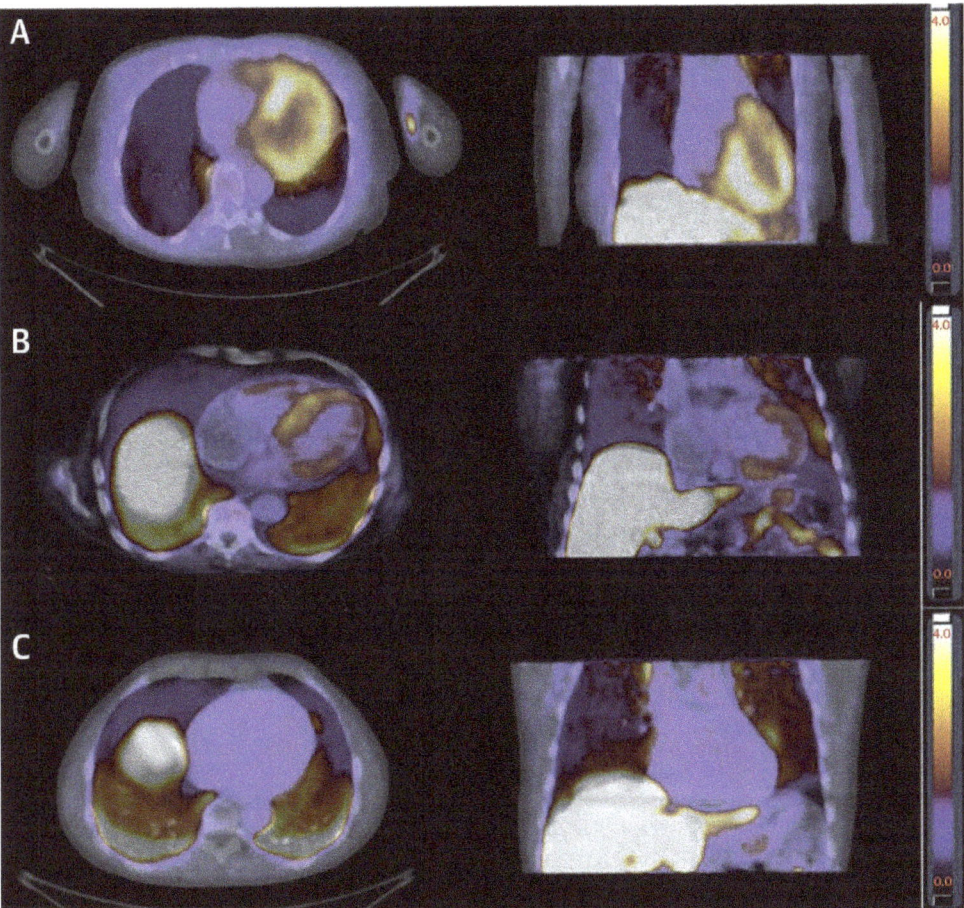

Figure 6. Examples of summed PET images taken 10–20 min after injection of ^{11}C-PIB (see below for abbreviations). The signal represents myocardium/blood SUV ratio, and the color scale ranges from black (SUV ratio 0) to white (SUV ratio 4.0). Transaxial and coronal view of (**A**) a patient with AL amyloidosis and high degree of ^{11}C-PIB uptake in the left ventricle wall and septum; (**B**) a patient with ATTR amyloidosis and moderate degree of ^{11}C-PIB uptake in the cardiac walls, most apparent in the septum; and (**C**) a healthy volunteer with no myocardial ^{11}C-PIB uptake. All subjects show high signal in the liver, which is due to normal metabolization of ^{11}C-PIB, and in the lungs, which is most likely caused by tracer lipophilicity. ATTR, transthyretin amyloidosis; PET, positron emission tomography; PIB, Pittsburgh compound B; SUV, standardized uptake value. Reproduced, with permission, from [50].

9. Cardiac Computed Tomography (CT)

The most powerful new imaging modality to emerge in the field of coronary artery disease is cardiac CT. Given a near perfect negative predictive value, it can exclude coronary disease with high reliability. The quantification of the severity of coronary stenoses is more difficult and fraught with the overestimation of the degree of stenosis, and further hampered by previous stent implantation. Artificial intelligence tools such as the available fractional flow reserve (CT-FFR) packages allow a rough non-invasive assessment of fractional flow reserve, but their clinical value is still under evaluation [51]. Apart from the diagnosis/exclusion of coronary artery disease, there is presently little role for CT in the routine workup of heart failure [52].

10. Pulmonary Hypertension

The evaluation of right ventricular systolic pressure is part of the standard echocardiographic examination, and, thus, the first step in the diagnostic work-up of suspected pulmonary hypertension. In the presence of pulmonary hypertension, echocardiography also allows to rule in or rule out left-sided diseases, such as valvular disease or LV systolic or diastolic dysfunction, as possible etiologies of pulmonary hypertension, although sometimes echocardiographic data are not conclusive, and invasive diagnostics by right-heart catheterization with exercise are necessary [53]. Furthermore, there is an overlap between classic primary pulmonary hypertension with normal pulmonary capillary wedge pressure and increased pulmonary vascular resistance on the one side and classic secondary pulmonary hypertension with increased wedge pressure and normal vascular resistance. Some patients show features of both categories, a condition termed "combined pre- and post-capillary pulmonary hypertension" [54]. Such "overlap" patients cannot be diagnosed with certainty using echocardiography alone, and need invasive workup.

11. How Should Cardiac Imaging Be Used "Wisely" in the Work-Up of Heart Failure?

Echocardiography remains the cornerstone of imaging in heart failure, and is considered mandatory by guidelines as an initial test. Apart from furnishing global functional measures of systolic and diastolic LV, as well as RV, function, echocardiography, in the majority of cases, detects probable underlying causes for heart failure, e.g., myocardial hypertrophy, infarct scars, valvular heart disease, and others. Nevertheless, echocardiography is often just the initial diagnostic step (see Table 1). Detailed information about myocardial structure and perfusion requires additional imaging tailored to the specific abnormalities and clinical circumstances. In this context, CMR allows (a limited) tissue characterization, and is strongly recommended by current heart failure guidelines "in selected cases", in particular with regard to the presence of myocarditis, storage diseases, iron overload/hemochromatosis, sarcoidosis, and certain cardiomyopathies such as hypertrophic, non-compaction, arrhythmogenic, and others [2]. Information about global and regional myocardial perfusion, including perfusion reserve, is available from CMR, SPECT, and PET, and may indicate the presence of epicardial coronary artery disease, microvascular disease, or another pathology.

Table 1. Goals, strengths, and limitations of cardiac imaging modalities in heart failure.

Modality	Goals	Strengths	Weaknesses/Limitations
Echocardiography	Measurement of systolic and diastolic function parameters (EF, GLS, etc.), identification of etiology (e.g., cardiomyopathies, coronary artery disease, hypertrophy, valvular heart disease)	Ubiquitous and prompt availability (first-line imaging modality for heart failure), good assessment of valvular heart disease, cost-effective, no side effects	High observer and test–retest variability, no tissue characterization, only indirect assessment of coronary artery disease by stress test, often limited by image quality
Cardiovascular Magnetic Resonance	Measurement of systolic and diastolic function parameters (LV and RV volumes, EF, GLS, etc.), identification of etiology of heart failure (ischemic scar, cardiomyopathy, myocarditis, storage disease, sarcoidosis, and others)	Tissue characterization by late enhancement and tissue relaxation parameters (T1, T2, T*); high volumetric accuracy (gold standard); ability to reliably quantify valvular regurgitation	Not everywhere available, expensive, limited in atrial fibrillation, some contraindications (renal failure for contrast application, some implanted devices, claustrophobia)
Cardiac Computed Tomography	Assessment of coronary artery disease; second-line imaging of structural disease (cardiomyopathies, valve disease)	Very high sensitivity for coronary artery disease; very high morphologic resolution	Radiation exposure, renal failure contraindication for contrast application

Table 1. Cont.

Modality	Goals	Strengths	Weaknesses/Limitations
Nuclear Perfusion Imaging	Assessment of myocardial perfusion (coronary or microvascular disease); assessment of amyloidosis with specific tracers; sarcoidosis	PET is gold standard for myocardial perfusion; identification of perfusion/metabolism mismatch, as in hibernating myocardium; high accuracy for amyloidosis and sarcoidosis; DPD imaging (planar/SPECT) is sensitive for cardiac ATTR amyloidosis	PET limited to centers with cyclotron; radiation exposure

12. Summary

Recent developments across all modalities of cardiac imaging have impacted the management of heart failure. The field has moved from just providing global information on LV performance, such as ejection fraction, to a multilayered diagnostic effort providing, in some cases, near-histologic diagnosis, and monitoring treatment success, e.g., the regression of amyloidosis [55]. Hence, it is important that the availability of modalities, as well as the competence in their application and interpretation, are safeguarded by professional and healthcare policies. A cooperative "cardiac imager team", bridging the gaps between cardiology, radiology, and nuclear medicine, is crucial to support the clinicians, and should be established in larger institutions. On the other hand, we must avoid the overuse of imaging, which is mostly due to a lack of a clear understanding of the strengths and weaknesses of particular modalities. A good example for such a strategy is the American College of Cardiology's "Choosing wisely" [56] campaign in cardiac imaging, and other bodies and countries should follow their example. Finally, it is important that imaging exams, if indicated, are performed with contemporary technology and interpretation skills in order to extract the maximum amount of useful information from each performed exam.

Funding: This research received no external funding.

Conflicts of Interest: The authors declare no conflict of interest.

References

1. Scholten, M.; Midlöv, P.; Halling, A. Disparities in prevalence of heart failure according to age, multimorbidity level and socioeconomic status in southern Sweden: A cross-sectional study. *BMJ Open* **2022**, *12*, e051997. [CrossRef] [PubMed]
2. McDonagh, T.A.; Metra, M.; Adamo, M.; Gardner, R.S.; Baumbach, A.; Böhm, M.; Burri, H.; Butler, J.; Čelutkienė, J.; Chioncel, O.; et al. 2021 ESC Guidelines for the diagnosis and treatment of acute and chronic heart failure. *Eur. Heart J.* **2021**, *42*, 3599–3726. [CrossRef]
3. Andersen, O.S.; Smiseth, O.A.; Dokainish, H.; Abudiab, M.M.; Schutt, R.C.; Kumar, A.; Sato, K.; Harb, S.; Gude, E.; Remme, E.W.; et al. Estimating left ventricular filling pressure by echocardiography. *J. Am. Coll. Cardiol.* **2017**, *69*, 1937–1948. [CrossRef]
4. Pak, M.; Kitai, T.; Kobori, A.; Sasaki, Y.; Okada, T.; Murai, R.; Toyota, T.; Kim, K.; Ehara, N.; Kinoshita, M.; et al. Diagnostic Accuracy of the 2016 Guideline-Based Echocardiographic Algorithm to Estimate Invasively-Measured Left Atrial Pressure by Direct Atrial Cannulation. *J. Am. Coll. Cardiol. Img.* **2022**, *15*, 1683–1691. [CrossRef] [PubMed]
5. Thavendiranathan, P.; Negishi, T.; Somerset, E.; Negishi, K.; Penicka, M.; Lemieux, J.; Aakhus, S.; Miyazaki, S.; Shirazi, M.; Galderisi, M.; et al. Strain-Guided Management of Potentially Cardiotoxic Cancer Therapy. *J. Am. Coll. Cardiol.* **2021**, *77*, 392–401. [CrossRef] [PubMed]
6. Kalam, K.; Otahal, P.; Marwick, T.H. Prognostic implications of global LV dysfunction: A systematic review and meta-analysis of global longitudinal strain and ejection fraction. *Heart* **2014**, *100*, 1673–1680. [CrossRef] [PubMed]
7. Inoue, K.; Khan, F.H.; Remme, E.W.; Ohte, N.; Garcıa-Izquierdo, E.; Chetrit, M.; Moñivas-Palomero, V.; Mingo-Santos, S.; Andersen, Ø.S.; Gude, E.; et al. Determinants of left atrial reservoir and pump strain and use of atrial strain for evaluation of left ventricular filling pressure. *Eur. Heart J. Cardiovasc. Imaging* **2021**, *23*, 61–70. [CrossRef] [PubMed]
8. Smiseth, O.A.; Morris, D.A.; Cardim, N.; Cikes, M.; Delgado, V.; Donal, E.; Flachskampf, F.A.; Galderisi, M.; Gerber, B.L.; Gimelli, A.; et al. Multimodality imaging in patients with heart failure and preserved ejection fraction: An expert consensus document of the European Association of Cardiovascular Imaging. *Eur. Heart J. Cardiovasc. Imaging* **2022**, *23*, e34–e61. [CrossRef]

9. Obokata, M.; Negishi, K.; Kurosawa, K.; Arima, H.; Tateno, R.; Ui, G.; Tange, S.; Arai, M.; Kurabayashi, M. Incremental diagnostic value of la strain with leg lifts in heart failure with preserved ejection fraction. *JACC Cardiovasc. Imaging* **2013**, *6*, 749–758. [CrossRef]
10. Yamada, H.; Kusunose, K.; Nishio, S.; Bando, M.; Hotchi, J.; Hayashi, S.; Ise, T.; Yagi, S.; Yamaguchi, K.; Iwase, T.; et al. Preload Stress Echocardiography Predicts Outcomes in Patients with Preserved Ejection Fraction and Low-Gradient Aortic Stenosis. *JACC Cardiovasc. Imaging* **2014**, *7*, 641–649. [CrossRef]
11. Tossavainen, E.; Wikström, G.; Henein, M.Y.; Lundqvist, M.; Wiklund, U.; Lindqvist, P. Passive leg-lifting in heart failure patients predicts exercise-induced rise in left ventricular filling pressures. *Clin. Res. Cardiol.* **2020**, *109*, 498–507. [CrossRef] [PubMed]
12. Helle-Valle, T.; Remme, E.W.; Lyseggen, E.; Pettersen, E.; Vartdal, T.; Opdahl, A.; Smith, H.J.; Osman, N.F.; Ihlen, H.; Edvardsen, T.; et al. Clinical assessment of left ventricular rotation and strain: A novel approach for quantification of function in infarcted myocardium and its border zones. *Am. J. Physiol. Heart Circ. Physiol.* **2009**, *297*, H257–H267. [CrossRef] [PubMed]
13. Villemain, O.; Correia, M.; Mousseaux, E.; Baranger, J.; Zarka, S.; Podetti, I.; Soulat, G.; Damy, T.; Hagège, A.; Tanter, M.; et al. Myocardial stiffness evaluation using noninvasive shear wave imaging in healthy and hypertrophic cardiomyopathic adults. *J. Am. Coll. Cardiovasc. Imaging* **2019**, *12*, 1135–1145. [CrossRef] [PubMed]
14. Villemain, O.; Baranger, J.; Friedberg, M.K.; Papadacci, C.; Dizeux, A.; Messas, E.; Tanter, M.; Pernot, M.; Mertens, L. Ultrafast Ultrasound Imaging in Pediatric and Adult Cardiology. Techniques, Applications, and Perspectives. *JACC Cardiovasc. Imaging* **2020**, *13*, 1771–1791. [CrossRef] [PubMed]
15. Doltra, A.; Bijnens, B.; Tolosana, J.M.; Borràs, R.; Khatib, M.; Penela, D.; De Caralt, T.M.; Castel, M.Á.; Berruezo, A.; Brugada, J.; et al. Mechanical abnormalities detected with conventional echocardiography are associated with response and midterm survival in CRT. *JACC Cardiovasc. Imaging* **2014**, *7*, 969–979. [CrossRef] [PubMed]
16. Baron, T.; Berglund, L.; Hedin, E.M.; Flachskampf, F.A. Test-retest reliability of new and conventional echocardiographic parameters of left ventricular systolic function. *Clin. Res. Cardiol.* **2019**, *108*, 355–365. [CrossRef] [PubMed]
17. Houard, L.; Militaru, S.; Tanaka, K.; Pasquet, A.; Vancraeynest, D.; Vanoverschelde, J.L.; Pouleur, A.C.; Gerber, B.L. Test-retest reliability of left and right ventricular systolic function by new and conventional echocardiographic and cardiac magnetic resonance parameters. *Eur. Heart J. Cardiovasc. Imaging* **2021**, *22*, 1157–1167. [CrossRef]
18. Kass, D.A.; Beyar, R. Evaluation of contractile state by maximal ventricular power divided by the square of end-diastolic volume. *Circulation* **1991**, *84*, 1698–1708. [CrossRef]
19. Harada, T.; Yamaguchi, M.; Omote, K.; Iwano, H.; Mizuguchi, Y.; Amanai, S.; Yoshida, K.; Kato, T.; Kurosawa, K.; Nagai, T.; et al. Cardiac Power Output Is Independently and Incrementally Associated with Adverse Outcomes in Heart Failure with Preserved Ejection Fraction. *Circ. Cardiovasc. Imaging* **2022**, *15*, e013495. [CrossRef]
20. Sörensen, J.; Harms, H.J.; Aalen, J.M.; Baron, T.; Smiseth, O.A.; Flachskampf, F.A. Myocardial Efficiency: A Fundamental Physiological Concept on the Verge of Clinical Impact. *JACC Cardiovasc. Imaging* **2020**, *13*, 1564–1576. [CrossRef] [PubMed]
21. Russell, K.; Eriksen, M.; Aaberge, L.; Wilhelmsen, N.; Skulstad, H.; Remme, E.W.; Haugaa, K.H.; Opdahl, A.; Fjeld, J.G.; Gjesdal, O.; et al. A novel clinical method for quantification of regional left ventricular pressure-strain loop area: A non-invasive index of myocardial work. *Eur. Heart J.* **2012**, *33*, 724–733. [CrossRef] [PubMed]
22. Aalen, J.M.; Donal, E.; Larsen, C.K.; Duchenne, J.; Lederlin, M.; Cvijic, M.; Hubert, A.; Voros, G.; Leclercq, C.; Bogaert, J.; et al. Imaging predictors of response to cardiac resynchronization therapy: Left ventricular work asymmetry by echocardiography and septal viability by cardiac magnetic resonance. *Eur. Heart J.* **2020**, *41*, 3813–3823. [CrossRef] [PubMed]
23. Smiseth, O.A.; Donal, E.; Penicka, M.; Sletten, O.J. How to measure ventricular myocardial work by pressure-strain loops. *Eur. Heart J. Cardiovasc. Imaging* **2021**, *22*, 259–261. [PubMed]
24. Truong, V.T.; Vo, H.Q.; Ngo, T.N.M.; Mazur, J.; Nguyen, T.T.H.; Pham, T.T.M.; Le, T.K.; Phan, H.; Palmer, C.; Nagueh, S.F.; et al. Normal Ranges of Global Left Ventricular Myocardial Work Indices in Adults: A Meta-Analysis. *J. Am. Soc. Echocardiogr.* **2022**, *35*, 369–377. [CrossRef] [PubMed]
25. Flachskampf, F.A.; Chandrashekar, Y. Myocardial work and myocardial work index: Relatives, but different. *JACC Cardiovascular. Imaging* **2022**, in press. [CrossRef]
26. Guazzi, M.; Bandera, F.; Pelissero, G.; Castelvecchio, S.; Menicanti, L.; Ghio, S.; Temporelli, P.L.; Arena, R. Tricuspid annular plane systolic excursion and pulmonary arterial systolic pressure relationship in heart failure: An index of right ventricular contractile function and prognosis. *Am. J. Physiol. Heart Circ. Physiol.* **2013**, *305*, H1373–H1381. [CrossRef] [PubMed]
27. Saeed, S.; Smith, J.; Grigoryan, K.; Lysne, V.; Rajani, R.; Chambers, J.B. The tricuspid annular plane systolic excursion to systolic pulmonary artery pressure index: Association with all-cause mortality in patients with moderate or severe tricuspid regurgitation. *Int. J. Cardiol.* **2020**, *317*, 176–180. [CrossRef] [PubMed]
28. Karam, N.; Stolz, L.; Orban, M.; Deseive, S.; Praz, F.; Kalbacher, D.; Westermann, D.; Braun, D.; Näbauer, M.; Neuss, M.; et al. Impact of Right Ventricular Dysfunction on Outcomes After Transcatheter Edge-to-Edge Repair for Secondary Mitral Regurgitation. *JACC Cardiovasc. Imaging* **2021**, *14*, 768–778. [CrossRef] [PubMed]
29. Karam, N.; Mehr, M.; Taramasso, M.; Besler, C.; Ruf, T.; Connelly, K.A.; Weber, M.; Yzeiraj, E.; Schiavi, D.; Mangieri, A.; et al. Value of Echocardiographic Right Ventricular and Pulmonary Pressure Assessment in Predicting Transcatheter Tricuspid Repair Outcome. *JACC Cardiovasc. Interv.* **2020**, *13*, 1251–1261. [CrossRef] [PubMed]

30. Lee, M.M.Y.; Brooksbank, K.J.M.; Wetherall, K.; Mangion, K.; Roditi, G.; Campbell, R.T.; Berry, C.; Chong, V.; Coyle, L.; Docherty, K.F.; et al. Effect of Empagliflozin on Left Ventricular Volumes in Patients with Type 2 Diabetes, or Prediabetes, and Heart Failure With Reduced Ejection Fraction (SUGAR-DM-HF). *Circulation* **2021**, *143*, 516–525. [CrossRef] [PubMed]
31. Dhingra, N.K.; Mistry, N.; Puar, P.; Verma, R.; Anker, S.; Mazer, C.D.; Verma, S. SGLT2 inhibitors and cardiac remodelling: A systematic review and meta-analysis of randomized cardiac magnetic resonance imaging trials. *ESC Heart Fail.* **2021**, *8*, 4693–4700. [CrossRef] [PubMed]
32. Sado, D.M.; White, S.K.; Piechnik, S.K.; Banypersad, S.M.; Treibel, T.; Captur, G.; Fontana, M.; Maestrini, V.; Flett, A.S.; Robson, M.D.; et al. Identification and assessment of Anderson-Fabry disease by cardiovascular magnetic resonance noncontrast myocardial T1 mapping. *Circ. Cardiovasc. Imaging* **2013**, *6*, 392–398. [CrossRef] [PubMed]
33. Phelan, D.; Collier, P.; Thavendiranathan, P.; Popović, Z.B.; Hanna, M.; Plana, J.C.; Marwick, T.H.; Thomas, J.D. Relative apical sparing of longitudinal strain using two-dimensional speckle-tracking echocardiography is both sensitive and specific for the diagnosis of cardiac amyloidosis. *Heart* **2012**, *98*, 1442–1448. [CrossRef] [PubMed]
34. Nitsche, C.; Scully, P.R.; Patel, K.P.; Kammerlander, A.A.; Koschutnik, M.; Dona, C.; Wollenweber, T.; Ahmed, N.; Thornton, G.D.; Kelion, A.D.; et al. Prevalence and Outcomes of Concomitant Aortic Stenosis and Cardiac Amyloidosis. *J. Am. Coll. Cardiol.* **2021**, *77*, 128–139. [CrossRef]
35. Puntmann, V.O.; Peker, E.; Chandrashekhar, Y.; Nagel, E. T1 Mapping in Characterizing Myocardial Disease: A Comprehensive Review. *Circ. Res.* **2016**, *119*, 277–299. [CrossRef]
36. Rodriguez-Granillo, G.A. Delayed enhancement cardiac computed tomography for the assessment of myocardial infarction: From bench to bedside. *Cardiovasc. Diagn. Ther.* **2017**, *7*, 159–170. [CrossRef]
37. Messroghli, D.R.; Moon, J.C.; Ferreira, V.M.; Grosse-Wortmann, L.; He, T.; Kellman, P.; Mascherbauer, J.; Nezafat, R.; Salerno, M.; Schelbert, E.B.; et al. Clinical recommendations for cardiovascular magnetic resonance mapping of T1, T2, T2* and extracellular volume: A consensus statement by the Society for Cardiovascular Magnetic Resonance (SCMR) endorsed by the European Association for Cardiovascular Imaging (EACVI). *J. Cardiovasc. Magn. Reson.* **2017**, *19*, 75.
38. Patel, A.R.; Kramer, C.M. Role of Cardiac Magnetic Resonance in the Diagnosis and Prognosis of Nonischemic Cardiomyopathy. *JACC Cardiovasc. Imaging* **2017**, *10 Pt A*, 1180–1193.
39. Haaf, P.; Garg, P.; Messroghli, D.R.; Broadbent, D.A.; Greenwood, J.P.; Plein, S. Cardiac T1 Mapping and Extracellular Volume (ECV) in clinical practice: A comprehensive review. *J. Cardiovasc. Magn. Reson.* **2016**, *18*, 89. [CrossRef]
40. Harries, I.; Berlot, B.; Ffrench-Constant, N.; Williams, M.; Liang, K.; De Garate, E.; Baritussio, A.; Biglino, G.; Plana, J.C.; Bucciarelli-Ducci, C. Cardiovascular magnetic resonance characterisation of anthracycline cardiotoxicity in adults with normal left ventricular ejection fraction. *Int. J. Cardiol.* **2021**, *343*, 180–186. [CrossRef]
41. Lisi, M.; Cameli, M.; Mandoli, G.E.; Pastore, M.C.; Righini, F.M.; D'Ascenzi, F.; Focardi, M.; Rubboli, A.; Mondillo, S.; Henein, M.Y. Detection of myocardial fibrosis by speckle-tracking echocardiography: From prediction to clinical applications. *Heart Fail. Rev.* **2022**. Epub ahead of print. [CrossRef] [PubMed]
42. Steeds, R.P.; Wheeler, R.; Bhattacharyya, S.; Reiken, J.; Nihoyannopoulos, P.; Senior, R.; Monaghan, M.J.; Sharma, V. Stress echocardiography in coronary artery disease: A practical guideline from the British Society of Echocardiography. *Echo Res. Pract.* **2019**, *6*, G17–G33. [CrossRef] [PubMed]
43. Shah, B.N.; Chahal, N.S.; Bhattacharyya, S.; Li, W.; Roussin, I.; Khattar, R.S.; Senior, R. The feasibility and clinical utility of myocardial contrast echocardiography in clinical practice: Results from the incorporation of myocardial perfusion assessment into clinical testing with stress echocardiography study. *J. Am. Soc. Echocardiogr.* **2014**, *27*, 520–530. [CrossRef] [PubMed]
44. Hsu, L.Y.; Groves, D.W.; Aletras, A.H.; Kellman, P.; Arai, A.E. A quantitative pixel-wise measurement of myocardial blood flow by contrast-enhanced first-pass CMR perfusion imaging: Microsphere validation in dogs and feasibility study in humans. *JACC Cardiovasc. Imaging* **2012**, *5*, 154–166. [CrossRef]
45. Arai, A.E.; Schulz-Menger, J.; Berman, D.; Mahrholdt, H.; Han, Y.; Bandettini, W.P.; Gutberlet, M.; Abraham, A.; Woodard, P.K.; Selvanayagam, J.B.; et al. Gadobutrol-enhanced magnetic resonance imaging for detection of coronary artery disease. *J. Am. Coll. Cardiol.* **2020**, *76*, 1536–1547. [CrossRef]
46. Kotecha, T.; Martinez-Naharro, A.; Boldrini, M. Automated pixel-wise quantitative myocardial perfusion mapping by CMR to detect obstructive coronary artery disease and coronary microvascular dysfunction. *J. Am. Coll. Cardiovasc. Imaging* **2019**, *12*, 1958–1969. [CrossRef]
47. Kotecha, T.; Chacko, L.; Chehab, O.; O'Reilly, N.; Martinez-Naharro, A.; Lazari, J.; Knott, K.D.; Brown, J.; Knight, D.; Muthurangu, V.; et al. Assessment of Multivessel Coronary Artery Disease Using Cardiovascular Magnetic Resonance Pixelwise Quantitative Perfusion Mapping. *JACC Cardiovasc. Imaging* **2020**, *13*, 2546–2557. [CrossRef]
48. Bonow, R.O.; Maurer, G.; Lee, K.L.; Holly, T.A.; Binkley, P.F.; Desvigne-Nickens, P.; Drozdz, J.; Farsky, P.S.; Feldman, A.M.; Doenst, T.; et al. Myocardial viability and survival in ischemic left ventricular dysfunction. *N. Engl. J. Med.* **2011**, *364*, 1617–1625. [CrossRef]
49. Almeida, A.G.; Carpenter, J.P.; Cameli, M.; Donal, E.; Dweck, M.R.; Flachskampf, F.A.; Maceira, A.M.; Muraru, D.; Neglia, D.; Pasquet, A.; et al. Multimodality imaging of myocardial viability: An expert consensus document from the European Association of Cardiovascular Imaging (EACVI). *Eur. Heart J. Cardiovasc. Imaging* **2021**, *22*, e97–e125. [CrossRef]

50. Rosengren, S.; Skibsted Clemmensen, T.; Tolbod, L.; Granstam, S.O.; Eiskjær, H.; Wikström, G.; Vedin, O.; Kero, T.; Lubberink, M.; Harms, H.J.; et al. Diagnostic Accuracy of [11C]PIB Positron Emission Tomography for Detection of Cardiac Amyloidosis. *JACC Cardiovasc. Imaging* **2020**, *13*, 1337–1347. [CrossRef]
51. Mathew, R.C.; Gottbrecht, M.; Salerno, M. Computed Tomography Fractional Flow Reserve to Guide Coronary Angiography and Intervention. *Interv. Cardiol. Clin.* **2018**, *7*, 345–354. [CrossRef] [PubMed]
52. Aziz, W.; Claridge, S.; Ntalas, I.; Gould, J.; de Vecchi, A.; Razeghi, O.; Toth, D.; Mountney, P.; Preston, R.; Rinaldi, C.A.; et al. Emerging role of cardiac computed tomography in heart failure. *ESC Heart Fail.* **2019**, *6*, 909–920. [CrossRef] [PubMed]
53. Humbert, M.; Kovacs, G.; Hoeper, M.M.; Badagliacca, R.; Berger, R.M.F.; Brida, M.; Carlsen, J.; Coats, A.J.S.; Escribano-Subias, P.; Ferrari, P.; et al. 2022 ESC/ERS Guidelines for the diagnosis and treatment of pulmonary hypertension. *Eur. Heart J.* **2022**. Online ahead of print. [CrossRef] [PubMed]
54. Maron, B.A.; Kovacs, G.; Vaidya, A.; Bhatt, D.L.; Nishimura, R.A.; Mak, S.; Guazzi, M.; Tedford, R.J. Cardiopulmonary Hemodynamics in Pulmonary Hypertension and Heart Failure: JACC Review Topic of the Week. *J. Am. Coll. Cardiol.* **2020**, *76*, 2671–2681. [CrossRef] [PubMed]
55. Fontana, M.; Martinez-Naharro, A.; Chacko, L.; Rowczenio, D.; Gilbertson, J.A.; Whelan, C.J.; Strehina, S.; Lane, T.; Moon, J.; Hutt, D.F.; et al. Reduction in CMR Derived Extracellular Volume with Patisiran Indicates Cardiac Amyloid Regression. *JACC Cardiovasc. Imaging* **2021**, *14*, 189–199. [CrossRef]
56. Available online: https://www.choosingwisely.org/societies/american-college-of-cardiology/ (accessed on 22 July 2022).

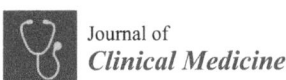

Systematic Review

Cardiomyopathy Associated with Right Ventricular Apical Pacing-Systematic Review and Meta-Analysis

Andrzej Osiecki [1,*], Wacław Kochman [1], Klaus K. Witte [2], Małgorzata Mańczak [3], Robert Olszewski [3,4] and Dariusz Michałkiewicz [1]

1. Department of Cardiovascular Diseases, Bielanski Hospital, Centre of Postgraduate Medical Education, Ceglowska 80 Street, 01-809 Warsaw, Poland
2. Leeds Institute of Cardiovascular and Metabolic Medicine, University of Leeds, Woodhouse Lane, Leeds LS2 9JT, UK
3. Department of Gerontology, Public Health and Didactics, National Institute of Geriatrics, Rheumatology and Rehabilitation in Warsaw, 1 Spartanska Street, 02-637 Warsaw, Poland
4. Department of Ultrasound, Institute of Fundamental Technological Research, Polish Academy of Sciences in Warsaw, 5B Pawinskiego Street, 02-106 Warsaw, Poland
* Correspondence: mcosiek@gmail.com; Tel.: +48-604138896

Abstract: AIMS: Bradyarrhythmias are potentially life-threatening medical conditions. The most widespread treatment for slow rhythms is artificial ventricular pacing. From the inception of the idea of artificial pacing, ventricular leads were located in the apex of the right ventricle. Right ventricular apical pacing (RVAP) was thought to have a deteriorating effect on left ventricular systolic function. The aim of this study was to systematically assess results of randomized controlled trials to determine the effects of right ventricular apical pacing on left ventricular ejection fraction (LVEF). Methods: we systematically searched the Cochrane Central Register of Controlled Trials, PubMed, and EMBASE databases for studies evaluating the influence of RVAP on LVEF. Pooled mean difference (MD) with a 95% confidence interval (CI) was estimated using a random effect model. Results: 14 randomized controlled trials (RCTs) comprising 885 patients were included. In our meta-analysis, RVAP was associated with statistically significant left ventricular systolic function impairment as measured by LVEF. The mean difference between LVEF at baseline and after intervention amounted to 3.35% (95% CI: 1.80–4.91). Conclusion: our meta-analysis confirms that right ventricular apical pacing is associated with progressive deterioration of left ventricular systolic function.

Keywords: artificial pacing; right ventricular pacing; left ventricular systolic function; heart failure

1. Introduction

Pacemaker implantation was a ground-breaking innovation in the history of medicine. Artificial pacing is the only successful treatment for patients with life-threatening bradyarrhythmias such as atrio-ventricular second/third degree blocks or symptomatic sinus node dysfunction. From the very beginning, the pacing electrode was implanted in the right ventricle. Over the course of time, right ventricular pacing (RVP) was suggested by several studies to be associated with an increased rate of newly appeared left ventricular dysfunction or with progression of pre-existing left ventricular dysfunction [1–3]. In the absence of the most credible type of evidence regarding the left ventricular systolic dysfunction associated with RVAP, we aimed to systematically evaluate the current literature and conduct a meta-analysis of randomized controlled trials (RCTs) and prospective studies comparing the mid- and long-term effects of right apical ventricular pacing on left ventricular systolic function as measured by left ventricular ejection fraction (LVEF).

2. Methods

2.1. Search Strategy

We systematically performed an electronic literature search of Cochrane Central Register of Controlled Trials, PubMed, and EMBASE databases from the time of database inception to October 2020 for studies evaluating the influence of RVAP on LVEF. We used search terms such as cardiomyopathy; heart failure; cardiac insufficiency; RV pacing; right ventricular pacing; artificial cardiac pacing; heart pacing; and artificial heart pacemaker during the search process. Reviews and reference lists of retrieved articles were hand searched for potentially relevant publications not previously identified in the database search. Our literature search was limited to prospective randomized trials published in peer-reviewed journals. All items resulting from these searches were reviewed at the title and abstract level and potentially eligible articles were reviewed in full text to assess eligibility. We also tried to obtain accessory information lacking in original articles through direct contact with the main authors.

2.2. Study Eligibility Criteria

We enrolled in our study prospective trials in which patients were at least 18 years old and underwent implantable cardioverter-defibrillator (ICD)/cardiac resynchronization therapy (CRT)/pacemaker implantation with pacing lead placement in the apex of the right ventricle. Because of statistical issues, cross-over trials needed to be excluded. Eligible studies had to report baseline LVEF and LVEF at the end of the follow-up or its change over the course of time. LVEF had to be assessed using echocardiography; trials in which LVEF was assessed using radionucleotide ventriculography were excluded from our analysis. Studies in which the RVAP percentage was absent or below 20% were excluded. Trials evaluating the effect of RVP after atrio-ventricular (AV) node ablation were also excluded. Studies in which a ventricular electrode was implanted in the right ventricular outflow tract or interventricular septum were not taken into consideration. Our analysis was limited to the groups of patients who were paced in synchronized atrio-univentricular mode or solely in univentricular mode (when the resynchronization device was implanted, the left ventricular lead had to be disactivated). We also limited our analysis to the trials in which the follow-up lasted at least 6 months.

2.3. Data Extraction

Independently, two investigators (A.O. and D.M.) extracted data from each eligible study, and potential disagreements were resolved by consensus. We documented the study characteristics (year of publication, study design, follow-up duration, and number of participants), patient demographics, and clinical characteristics (type of underlying cardiomyopathy, presence of hypertension, diabetes mellitus, coronary artery disease, or prior myocardial infarction with concomitant atrial fibrillation). We also extracted information about baseline LVEF, LVEF at the end of the follow-up, or differences between these two values.

2.4. Statistical Analysis

Pooled mean difference (MD) with a 95% confidence interval (CI) was estimated using a random effect model. Heterogeneity of the studies was determined using an inconsistency index I^2 (0–100%) and between-study variance of true effects T^2. An I^2 value higher than 50% indicates substantial heterogeneity, and a value higher than 75% indicates high heterogeneity. A $T^2 > 0$ is considered substantial. To assess the influence of each individual study on the overall result of the meta-analysis, a sensitivity analysis was performed, which consisted of removing the individual study from the calculations. Publication bias was evaluated using a funnel plot with the Begg–Mazumdar and Egger test and the Cochrane risk of bias tool for randomized trials (RoB 2). To assess the influence of individual studies on the meta-analysis, calculations were repeated excluding one of the studies. A p-value of less than 0.05 was considered significant. All statistical analyses were carried out using STATISTICA v.13.1 (Dell Inc. 2016, Tulsa, OK, USA).

3. Results

The systematic review and meta-analysis were performed according to the Preferred Reporting Items for Systematic Reviews and Meta-Analyses (PRISMA) statement for reporting systematic reviews and meta-analyses of RCTs. Our literature search identified 574 studies (Figure 1). After the exclusion of duplicates and non-relevant studies, 36 studies were retrieved for further full-text evaluation by reviewing study titles and abstracts. We further excluded three studies that were projected in cross-over manner [4–6], six trials that did not evaluate LVEF in the follow-up [7–12], seven studies in which information about RVAP was absent or RVAP was <20% [13–19], three studies in which patients were treated according to the "ablate and pace" method [20–22], one trial with a short-term follow-up [23], one trial which was a prolonged follow-up of the so far included study, and one study because of statistical issues [24]. Finally, fourteen randomized controlled studies published in the period of 2008–2017 were included in this systematic review and meta-analysis.

Study and patient characteristics are summarized in Table 1. The eligible studies included a total of 885 patients. Study participants were predominantly male (ranging from 30% to 72.8% male), and their mean age ranged from 67.1 to 77 years. The apical location of the ventricular pacing electrode was defined in 13 studies; in the Block HF study, the pacing/defibrillating electrode was placed in the apex in the majority of patients (211/342). The mean follow-up in the included studies ranged between 6 and 89 months.

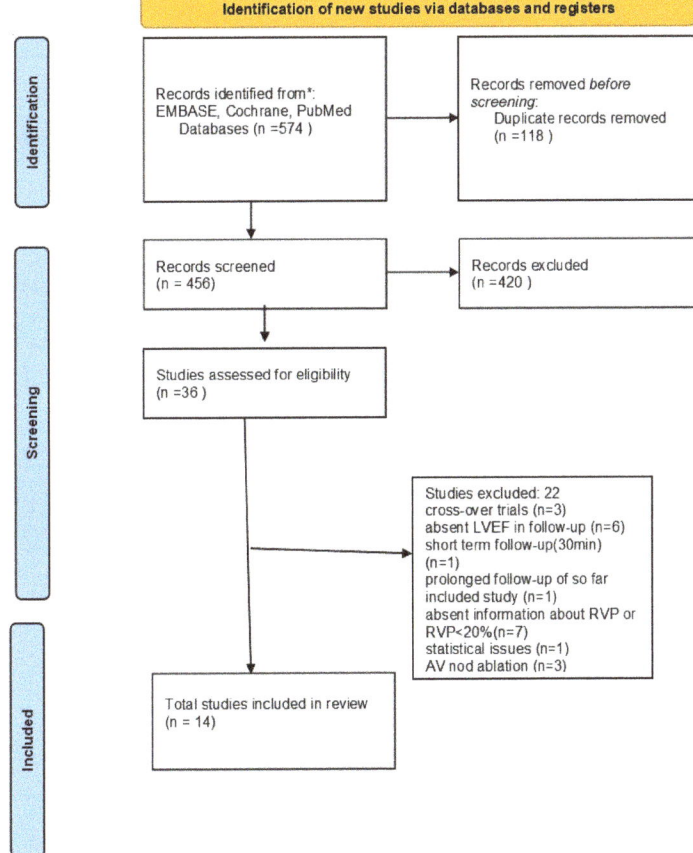

Figure 1. PRISMA flow diagram.

Table 1. Studies and patient characteristics.

Author (Year)	Title	Reason for Cardiac Implantable Electronic Device (CIED) Implantation	Primary Pacing Mode in Analysed Group	Right Ventricular Lead Location in Analysed Group	Study Design	Observation Period (Months)	Subjects, n	Men, n (%)	Age, Mean (SD) (Years)	RV Pacing (%)	Baseline LVEF (%) (SD)	LVEF in Follow-Up (%) (SD)	Baseline Mean QRS Duration, (ms)	Paced QRS Duration (ms)	Baseline LVEDD (mm)	Follow-Up LVEDD (mm)	Baseline LVEDV (mL)	Follow-Up LVEDV (mL)	Baseline LVESV (mL)	Follow-Up LVESV (mL)
St. John Sutton et al. (2015) * [25]	Reverse Remodeling with Biventricular Pacing	Atrio-ventricular block in patients with heart failure in NYHA functional class I-III and LVEF ≤ 50%	DDD(R)/VVI(R)	Apical position (211/342) Other than apical position within RV (131/342)	Multicenter, prospective, randomized, double blinded trial	24	342	249 (72.8)	73.0 ± 10.6	98.6-AVB 3d-167 patients 97.8-AVB 2d-108 patients 97-AVB 1d-66 patients	33.6 ± 9.2	−1.6% (95% CI), SD 10,499	123 ± 30.8	NA	CRT-P RVP 53 ± 8 CRT-D RVP 54 ± 7	CRT-P RV 53 ± 7.9 CRT-D RV 57 ± 8.27	189.2 ± 64.0	188.0 ± 66.8	127.9 ± 53.1	129.8 ± 58.7
Albertsen AE. et al. (2008) [26]	DDD(R) pacing, but not AAI(R) pacing induces left ventricular desynchronization in patients with sick sinus syndrome and tissue-Doppler and 3D echocardiographic evaluation in a randomized controlled comparison	Patients with sick sinus syndrome with either syncope or dizzy spell or heart failure and electrocardiographic abnormalities; sinus arrest > 2 s or tachy-brady syndrome with sinus pauses > 2 s or sinus bradycardia < 40 bpm in awake hours	DDD(R)	Apical position	Single-center, prospective, randomized trial	12	26	8 (30)	73 ± 13	66	63.1 ± 8	59.3 ± 8	NA	NA	NA	NA	NA	NA	NA	NA
Yu C.M. et al. (2009) [27]	Biventricular pacing in patients with bradycardia and normal ejection fraction (PACE).	Patients with sinus node dysfunction or bradycardia due to advanced atrioventricular block and normal ejection fraction(45%)	DDDR	Apical position	Multicenter, prospective, double blind, randomized trial	12	88	49 (56)	68 ± 11	97	61.5 ± 6.6	54.8 ± 9.1	107 ± 30	NA	NA	NA	73.3 ± 19.8	76.7 ± 22.5	28.6 ± 10.7	35.7 ± 16.3
Gierula J. et al. (2013) [28]	Cardiac resynchronization therapy in pacemaker-dependent patients with left ventricular dysfunction.	Patients with implanted pacemaker, unavoidable RV pacing > 80%, reduced LVEF < 50% listed for routine pacemaker replacement due to battery depletion	DDD(R)/VVI(R)	Apical position	Single-center, prospective, randomized, unblinded trial	6	25	16 (64)	77 ± 4	98.34 ± 3.47	41 ± 4 (37–45) 95% CI	39.75 ± 8.27	159 ± 10	NA	49.2 ± 3	NA	NA	NA	NA	NA
XU H. et al. (2017) [29]	Early Right Ventricular Apical Pacing-Induced Gene Expression Alterations Are Associated with Deterioration of Left Ventricular Systolic Function: Dis Markers	Patients with complete atrioventricular block and preserved LVEF ≥ 50%	DDD(R)	Apical position	Single-center, prospective randomized controlled trial	24	30	17 (56.7)	67.1 ± 7.5	100	63.0 ± 5.4	56.7 ± 7.6	102 ± 11	154 ± 12	NA	NA	103.2 ± 11.4	NA	37.8 ± 5.1	NA

32

Table 1. Cont.

Author (Year)	Title	Reason for Cardiac Implantable Electronic Device (CIED) Implantation	Study Design	Observation Period (Months)	Subjects, n	Men, n (%)	Age, Mean (SD) (Years)	RV Pacing (%)	Baseline LVEF (%) (SD)	LVEF in Follow-Up (%) (SD)	Baseline Mean QRS Duration, (ms)	Paced QRS Duration (ms)	Baseline LVEDD (mm)	Follow-Up LVEDD (mm)	Baseline LVEDV (mL)	Follow-Up LVEDV (mL)	Baseline LVESV (mL)	Follow-Up LVESV (mL)
Mitov VM, et al. (2016) [30]	The Effect of Right Ventricular Pacemaker Lead Position on Functional Status in Patients with Preserved Left Ventricular Ejection Fraction	Patients with preserved EF ≥ 54% and indication for antibradycardia pacing	DDDR)/VVI(R)	Apical position	Single-center, prospective, randomized trial	12	61	43 (70.5)	72.72 ± 9.4	68.55 ± 39.34	59.16 ± 10.43	60.96 ± 10.56	91.15 ± 20.33	151.34	NA	NA	NA	NA	NA	NA
Kaye, G. C. et al. (2015) [31]	Effect of right ventricular pacing lead site on left ventricular function in patients with high-grade atrioventricular block: results of the Protect-Pace study	Patients with persistent 2:1 atrio-ventricular block or permanent AF and sinus rhythm and heart block with LVEF ≥ 40% and no clinical signs of heart failure	DDDR)/VVI(R)	Apical position	Multicenter prospective randomized, trial	24	120	73 (60.8)	73.7 ± 11.1	98 ± 11	57 ± 9	55 ± 9	NA	NA	NA	NA	NA	NA	NA	NA
Molina L. et al. (2013) [32]	Medium-Term Effects of Septal and Apical Pacing in Pacemaker-Dependent Patients: A Double-Blind Prospective Randomized Study	Patients with complete heart block with no evidence of severe heart failure (NYHA IV).	DDDR)	Apical position	Single-center, prospective randomized double-blind trial	24	34	14 (40.3)	72 ± 12	≥98	52 ± 10	54 ± 11	NA	NA	50 ± 8	46.9 ± 6.2	70.6 ± 34.0	61.9 ± 22.2	35.6 ± 27.1	31.8 ± 20.7
Lewicka-Nowak E. et al. (2006) [33]	Right ventricular apex versus right ventricular outflow tract pacing: prospective, randomised, long-term clinical and echocardiographic evaluation.	Patients with indications for permanent pacing, who required VDD, DDD or VVI/R pacemaker implantation.	VDD/DDD/VVI(R)	Apical position	Single-center prospective, randomised trial	89 ± 9	14	7 (50)	76 ± 9	94 ± 13	56 ± 11	47 ± 8	NA	QRS duration at the initial examination: 154 ± 16 QRS duration at the end of follow up: 178 ± 19	49 ± 6	49 ± 8	NA	NA	NA	NA
Zhang HX, et al. (2012) [34]	Comparison of right ventricular outflow tract septum pacing and right ventricular apex pacing in the elderly with normal left ventricular ejection fraction: long-term follow-up.	Patients between 65 to 85 years of age with conventional pacing indications for permanent pacing, no clinical manifestations of congestive heart failure (HF) and chronic renal insufficiency, without diagnosed AF prior to pacemaker implantation	DDDR)	Apical position	Single-centre prospective, randomised trial	31.5 (13–58)	32	18 (56)	75 ± 10	82.91 ± 13.32	59.5 ± 6.21	54.22 ± 8.73	106.25 ± 18.36	143.56 ± 12.90	47.16 ± 3.63	49.22 ± 5.16	NA	NA	NA	NA

Table 1. *Cont.*

Author (Year)	Title	Reason for Cardiac Implantable Electronic Device (CIED) Implantation	Primary Pacing Mode in Analysed Group	Right Ventricular Lead Location in Analysed Group	Study Design	Observation Period (Months)	Subjects, n	Men, n (%)	Age, Mean (SD) (Years)	RV Pacing (%)	Baseline LVEF (%) (SD)	LVEF in Follow-Up (%) (SD)	Baseline Mean QRS Duration, (ms)	Paced QRS Duration (ms)	Baseline LVEDD (mm)	Follow-Up LVEDD (mm)	Baseline LVEDV (mL)	Follow-Up LVEDV (mL)	Baseline LVESV (mL)	Follow-Up LVESV (mL)
Flevari P. et al. (2009) [35]	Long-term nonoutflow tract septal versus apical right ventricular pacing: relation to left ventricular dyssynchrony.	Patients with persistent first-degree AV block, a relatively long PR interval (PR > 280 ms), a sinus rate > 60 bpm, and intermittent second- or third-degree AV block.	DDD(R)	Apical position	Single-center, prospective, randomised, trial	12	15	9 (60)	72 ± 1.5	97 ± 5	49 ± 4.3 On intrinsic rhythm	43 ± 3.1 On paced rhythm	153 ± 5.1	171 ± 4.5	NA	NA	85 ± 4.9	96 ± 5.2	39 ± 4.0	43 ± 3.0
Gong X. et al. (2009) [36]	Is right ventricular outflow tract pacing superior to right ventricular apex pacing in patients with normal cardiac function?	Patients with high or complete atrio-ventricular block, LVEF > 50% and no clinical signs of congestive heart failure necessitating permanent pacemaker implantation.	DDD(R)	Apical position	Single-center, prospective, randomized trial	12	44	25 (57)	70 ± 11	97.3	67.92 ± 6.38	65.71 ± 6.56	97.23 ± 8.89	177.14 ± 22.52	NA	NA	84.32 ± 22.05	78.45 ± 17.91	27.23 ± 9.54	26.70 ± 9.54
Cano O. et al. (2010) [37]	Comparison of effectiveness of right ventricular septal pacing versus right ventricular apical pacing.	Patients with an indication for permanent cardiac pacing because of atrioventricular block or sick sinus syndrome, with no sings of heart failure and LVEF ≥ 50%.	DDD/VVI	Apical position	Single-center prospective randomized, single-blind,	12	28	14 (50)	72 ± 10	88.4 ± 17.1	62.9 ± 6.3 On paced rhythm	62.9 ± 7.9 On paced rhythm	NA	NA	NA	NA	88.6 ± 24.3	79.5 ± 29.8	33.2 ± 12.9	30.1 ± 14.5
Leong DF et al. (2010) [38]	Long-term mechanical consequences of permanent right ventricular pacing: effect of pacing site.	Patients with conventional indications for pacemaker implantation(SSS; AVB) without indications for cardiac resynchronization therapy.	DDD	Apical position	Double-center prospective, randomized trial	30 ± 12	26	16 (61)	77 ± 8	49 ± 42	60 ± 6 On paced rhythm	52 ± 9 On paced rhythm	NA	156 ± 21	NA	NA	NA	88 ± 39	NA	45 ± 26

* Discrepancies in baseline LVEF between an article witten by Curtis and paper written by Sutton, both of them being based on the same Block HF Study, derive from different data collection methods. Curtis used data reported by the sites on the patient history form. Sutton, on other hand, used data measured by the echo core lab. LVEF—left ventricular ejection fraction; LVEDD—left ventricular end-diastolic diameter; LVESD—left ventricular end-systolic diameter; LVEDV—left ventricular end-diastolic volume; LVESV—left ventricular end-systolic volume; NA—not available.

3.1. Risk of Bias

Using a revised Cochrane risk of bias tool for randomized trials (RoB 2), risk of bias of the included studies was estimated (Figure 2.)

Intention-to-treat	Unique ID	Study ID	Experimental	Comparator	Outcome	Weight	D1	D2	D3	D4	D5	Overall		
	PICM-2022	Yu CM(2009)	NA	NA	LVEF	1	+	+	+	+	+	+	+	Low risk
	PICM-2022	Albertsen AE(2008)	NA	NA	LEVF	1	!	+	+	+	+	!	!	Some concerns
	PICM-2022	St. John Sutton(2015)	NA	NA	LVEF	1	+	+	!	+	+	!	−	High risk
	PICM-2022	Gierula J.(2013)	NA	NA	LVEF	1	!	+	+	+	+	!		
	PICM-2022	Mitov(2016)	NA	NA	LVEF	1	!	+	+	−	!	−	D1	Randomisation process
	PICM-2022	Kaye G.(2015)	NA	NA	LVEF	1	+	+	+	+	+	+	D2	Deviations from the intended interventions
	PICM-2022	Lewicka-Nowak E.(2006)	NA	NA	LVEF	1	!	!	!	−	!	−	D3	Missing outcome data
	PICM-2022	Zhang HX.(2012)	NA	NA	LVEF	1	!	+	+	+	!	!	D4	Measurement of the outcome
	PICM-2022	Flevari P.(2009)	NA	NA	LVEF	1	+	+	+	−	!	−	D5	Selection of the reported result
	PICM-2022	Gong X.(2009)	NA	NA	LVEF	1	!	!	+	+	!	!		
	PICM-2022	Cano O.(2010)	NA	NA	LVEF	1	!	+	!	!	!	!		
	PICM-2022	Leong DP.(2010)	NA	NA	LVEF	1	!	!	−	+	!	−		
	PICM-2022	Xu H.(2017)	NA	NA	LVEF	1	+	!	+	+	+	!		
	PICM-2022	Molina L.(2013)	NA	NA	LVEF	1	!	+	+	!	+	!		

Figure 2. Risk of bias summary for the included studies. Green indicates low risk of bias. Red indicates high risk of bias. Yellow indicates some concerns [25–38].

3.2. Echocardiographic Changes

(a) LVEF. The mean difference between LVEF at baseline and after intervention amounted to 3.35% (95% CI: 1.80–4.91). A forrest plot of pooled differences is presented in Figure 3. There was substantial heterogeneity among the included studies: $I^2 = 72.1$ (95% CI: 52.2–83.7) and $T^2 = 5.6$ (95% CI: 2.4–11.0). The sensitivity analysis showed no significant changes in the overall result of the meta-analysis. When excluding individual studies from the calculations, the overall result was still above 3 and ranged from 3.01 (95% CI: 1.49–4.53) to 3.72 (95% CI: 2.19–5.26). No relationship has been found between effect sizes and standard errors: Begg–Mazumdar test; $p = 0.625$, Egger test; $p = 0.775$.

(b) LVESV. Six studies reported results regarding change in LVESV during the course of the trial. The overall mean difference in LVESV equalled −2.09 mL (95% CI: −5.30–1.13), indicating no significant change of LVESV after RVP. There was moderate heterogeneity across studies ($I^2 = 57.19\%$; 95% CI: 0.00–82.72%). The exclusion of individual articles did not significantly change the overall result. It was still statistically insignificant and ranged from −0.92 (95% CI: −4.12–2.28) to −2.91 (95% CI: −6.43–0.61).

(c) LVEDV. Six studies reported results regarding change in LVEDV during the course of the trial. The mean difference in LVEDV was 0.45 mL (95% CI: −7.05–7.45), indicating a lack of RVP influence on LVEDV. There was substantial heterogeneity across studies ($I^2 = 80.89\%$; 95% CI: 58.88–91.12%). The exclusion of individual studies did not change the overall result significantly. It ranged from -0.89 (95% CI: −8.71–6.93) to 2.50 (95% CI: −2.62–7.62).

(d) 6 min walk test (6MWT). Six studies reported result of 6 min walk test both initially and at the end of the follow-up. The pooled mean difference was −26.93 m, which means that RVAP was associated with an increase in 6MWT after the intervention (Figure 4.). There was substantial heterogeneity across studies ($I^2 = 44.99\%$, 95% CI: 0.00–79.83%). The sensitivity analysis showed no significant changes in the overall 6MWT result. When excluding individual studies from the calculations, the range of values was from −21.04 (95% CI: −41.89–0.20) to −38.99 (95% CI: −61.14–16.85).

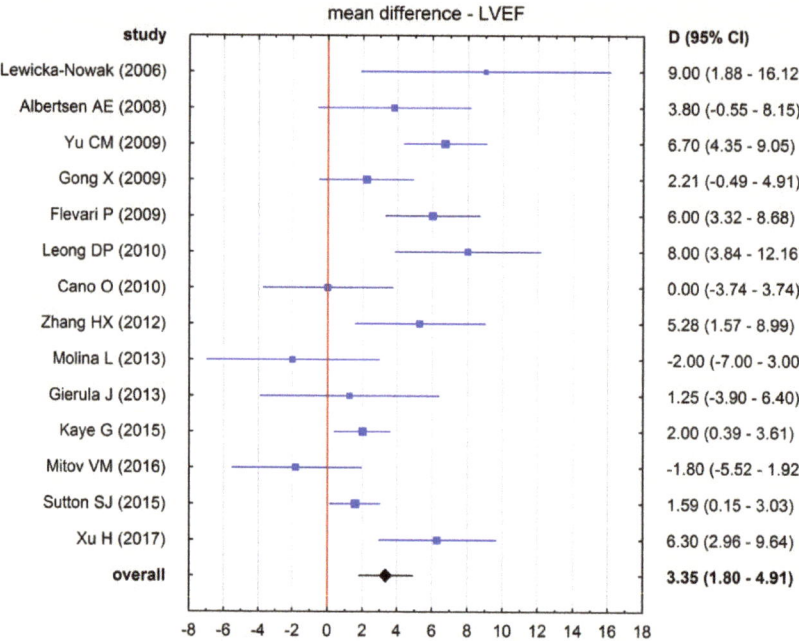

Figure 3. Forrest plot illustrating pooled mean difference (MD) with a 95% confidence interval (CI) of LVEF (%) [25–38].

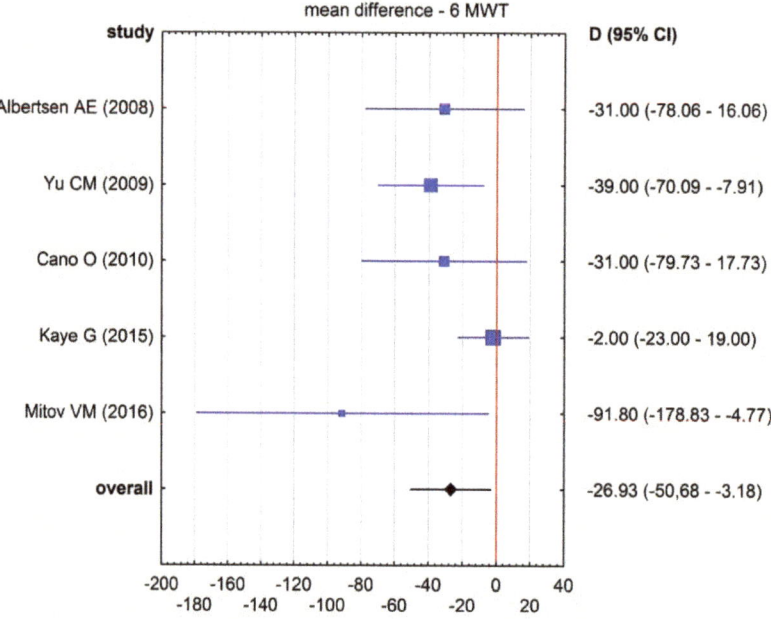

Figure 4. Forrest plot illustrating pooled mean difference (MD) with a 95% confidence interval (CI) of 6MWT (meters) [26,27,30,31,37].

4. Discussion

To the best of our knowledge, this is the first study to analyze the influence of right ventricular apical pacing on LVEF in patients with dominant sinus rhythm and to comprise only prospective randomized trials. The result of our meta-analysis confirms that RVAP is associated with continuous deterioration of the left ventricular systolic function.

One of the most important factors predisposing individuals to LV systolic dysfunction is a substantial percentage of RVAP. Systolic function impairment measured by a shortening fraction in the setting of a high percentage of RVP (90%) was seen in the DDDR group in the study comparing AAIR and DDDR pacing in patients with sick sinus syndrome [39]. In the study conducted by Gierula et al., investigators reprogrammed pacemakers to minimize RVP in patients with avoidable RVP. After six months of follow-up, they obtained a mean of 49% reduction in RVP with simultaneous LVEF improvement at the level of 6% [40]. In the ANSWER trial, in which the SafeR strategy was implemented to reduce RVP in the general pacemaker population, it was shown that this tool was effective in RVP reduction in comparison to typical DDD pacing, although it did not have an overall effect on the composite primary end point (hospitalization for heart failure (HF), atrial fibrillation (AF), or cardioversion). However, it is worth mentioning that in this trial, HF hospitalizations showed a trend favouring SafeR [41]. Regarding the PreFER MVP trial, despite a reduction in RVP through the use of MVP (Managed Ventricular Pacing) mode, it did not lead to clinical benefits in terms of cardiovascular (CV) hospitalizations, death, or permanent or persistent AF [42]. Finally, Kiehl et al. concluded that, in populations with complete heart block and preimplant preserved LVEF, a right ventricular pacing burden of $\geq 20\%$ was strongly associated with the development of PICM (Pacemaker induced cardiomyopathy) [43].

Another factor which might influence susceptibility to "pacing"-induced HF is the degree of left ventricular systolic dysfunction at the time of pacemaker implantation. In the DANPACE study, in which AAIR pacing was compared to DDDR pacing in patients with sick sinus syndrome (SSS) and preserved left ventricular systolic function (mean follow-up of 5.4 ± 2.6 years), no difference related to hospitalizations for HF, New York Heart Association functional class, or use of diuretics was found, despite a high percentage of ventricular stimulation in DDDR group ($65 \pm 33\%$) [11]. On the other hand, the study conducted by Albertsen et al. found LVEF deterioration in patients with preserved systolic function, a third-degree AV block, and DDDR pacemaker implantation, although this result did not yield change in functional status. Notably, in this trial, the ventricular electrode was implanted in the right ventricular outflow tract [44]. A similar result was reported by Crevelari; in her research, no hospitalization due to heart failure was observed. However, 23.5% of patients with RVP had over 10% LVEF reduction at the end of the follow-up [7]. According to the three meta-analyses, right ventricular non-apical electrode location ensures less harmful influence on LVEF in comparison with its apical location [45–47].

According to the DAVID (Dual-Chamber Pacing or Ventricular Backup Pacing in Patients With an Implantable Defibrillator) trial, the DDDR pacing mode appeared to be disadvantageous for patients with reduced EF (mean LVEF 40% or less), typical indications for an ICD, and no necessity for antibradycardia pacing [3]. The population of patients with reduced EF and prior MI was also investigated in the MADIT II trial, in which patients were either protected with ICD with antibradycardia ventricular backup pacing or continued conventional pharmacological therapy [48]. The authors of this study reported the concerning observation that patients treated with ICD had to be hospitalized more frequently due to new or worsened heart failure.

Additional insight into PICM (pacemaker-induced cardiomyopathy) came from retrospective analysis of the MOST trial. Sweeney et al. suggested that pacemaker-induced cardiomyopathy is a complex medical entity dependent on "play" between substrates and promoters. Substrates were described as specific clinical and physiological variables present at the pre-implantation stage, such as atrial rhythm, AV conduction, ventricular conduction, ventricular function, symptomatic heart failure, and prior myocardial infarction (MI).

Promoters were directly associated with pacemaker implantation and postimplantation parameters, including ventricular desynchronization (paced QRS duration and cumulative %VP) and AV desynchronization (pacing mode). Surprisingly, not only prolonged postimplantation paced QRS duration but also prolonged postimplantation spontaneous QRS duration increased the risk of heart failure development, especially in patients with history of MI and low EF [49]. In our analysis, we were not able to systematically assess the influence of postimplantation paced QRS duration on LVEF because of insufficient data.

We suspect that pacing duration has substantial importance for PICM development. The longest duration of follow-up in the trials included in our meta-analysis was 89 months. In the long-term follow-up of patients included in the PACE trial, which lasted almost 5 years, investigators observed a significant LVEF reduction (62.0 $\pm$ 6.3% vs. 53.2 $\pm$ 8.2%) with a simultaneously maintained high RVP percentage (94.5 $\pm$ 19.5%) [24]. The follow-up duration in most of the aforementioned trials lasted up to 5 years [11]. Therefore, we cannot exclude that systolic dysfunction appears or accelerates after this period of time.

Our analysis showed no relationship between RVP and changes in LVESV or LVEDV.

The result of the 6MWT analysis was surprising is. Almost all studies included patients with preserved EF, except for one (Kaye et al.) in which patients' LVEF was at least 40%, but no clinical signs and symptoms were observed. Four studies (Albertsen, Kaye, Yu, and Gong) reported deterioration of LVEF during the follow-up. Intuitively, a dependence between LVEF and the distance covered in the 6MWT would be expected. However, according to the literature, there is no correlation between systolic function and distance covered in the 6MWT in patients with heart failure [50,51]. A partial explanation for abovementioned result is chronotropic incompetence and atrio-ventricular conduction impairment, which were primary indicators for antibradycardia pacing in the analyzed studies. Sinus node dysfunction and atrio-ventricular conduction disabilities might be responsible for an insufficient cardiovascular response to exercise tolerance tests.

Ordinary right ventricular pacing is less expensive and less time consuming in comparison with innovative types of pacing such as resynchronization therapy or conducting system pacing. Whenever unfavourable effects of RVP are more probable (prospective high percentage of ventricular pacing, symptomatic heart failure, or young patient age), strategies other than RV apical pacing should be considered.

Limitations

In the study conducted by Gierula et al., the patients included in the trial were already pacemaker dependent (unavoidable RVP > 80%), and they had been paced for at least 10 years before pacemaker replacement. Based upon this information, we cannot estimate the real influence of RV pacing on left ventricular systolic function, as their LVEF might have already been impaired due to substantial pacing percentages [28]. Our focus was to evaluate apical pacing, but we included one study in which the pacing/defibrillating electrode was located within the right ventricle but not in the RV apex in the minority of participants (131/342), which might influence the results of our study [25]. In studies conducted by Leong, Cano, Lewicka-Nowak, and Molina, baseline echocardiography examinations were made on active pacing, which might have influenced initial LVEF measurements [32,33,37,38]. Significant differences in follow-up duration among studies (from 6 months to 89 months) also emerged as a limitation of this study. We cannot completely exclude that LVEF at the end of the follow-up was biased by conditions having significant influence on left ventricular systolic function (such as myocardial infarction or myocarditis), but it would be rather unusual that these co-morbidities would have changed results of 14 randomized controlled trials and obscured real effects of RVAP on LVEF. We could not accurately analyze pre-implantation data influencing LVEF deterioration because of their incompleteness.

5. Conclusions

Our meta-analysis confirmed that right ventricular apical pacing is associated with progressive deterioration of left ventricular systolic function. The association between RVP and LV systolic function deterioration was particularly observed in patients with high RVP percentage. Before pacemaker implantation, baseline patient characteristics always need to be collected in order to properly qualify patients for intervention and avoid adverse effects of apical pacing in the future.

Author Contributions: Conceptualization: A.O. and D.M.; methodology: A.O. and R.O.; software: M.M.; validation: A.O., D.M. and W.K.; formal analysis: A.O.; investigation: A.O. and D.M.; resources: A.O. and D.M.; data curation: A.O. and D.M.; writing—original draft preparation: A.O.; writing—review and editing: D.M. and W.K.; supervision: K.K.W.; project administration: A.O. All authors have read and agreed to the published version of the manuscript.

Funding: This research received no external funding.

Institutional Review Board Statement: Not applicable.

Informed Consent Statement: Not applicable.

Data Availability Statement: Direct contact with main author, A.O., e-mail: mcosiek@gmail.com.

Conflicts of Interest: The authors declare no conflict of interest.

References

1. Khurshid, S.; Epstein, A.E.; Verdino, R.J.; Lin, D.; Goldberg, L.R.; Marchlinski, F.E.; Frankel, D.S. Incidence and predictors of right ventricular pacing-induced cardiomyopathy. *Heart Rhythm* **2014**, *11*, 1619–1625. [CrossRef]
2. Zhang, X.-H.; Chen, H.; Siu, C.-W.; Yiu, K.-H.; Chan, W.-S.; Lee, K.L.; Chan, H.-W.; Lee, S.W.; Fu, G.-S.; Lau, C.-P.; et al. New-Onset Heart Failure After Permanent Right Ventricular Apical Pacing in Patients with Acquired High-Grade Atrioventricular Block and Normal Left Ventricular Function. *J. Cardiovasc. Electrophysiol.* **2007**, *19*, 136–141. [CrossRef] [PubMed]
3. The DAVID Trial Investigators. Dual-Chamber Pacing or Ventricular Backup Pacing in Patients With an Implantable Defibrillator: The Dual Chamber and VVI Implantable Defibrillator (DAVID) Trial. *JAMA* **2002**, *288*, 3115–3123. [CrossRef]
4. Chwyczko, T.; Dąbrowski, R.; Maciąg, A.; Sterlinski, M.; Smolis-Bąk, E.; Borowiec, A.; Kowalik, I.; Łabęcka, A.; Jankowska, A.; Kośmicki, M.; et al. Potential Prevention of Pacing-Induced Heart Failure Using Simple Pacemaker Programming Algorithm. *Ann. Noninvasive Electrocardiol.* **2013**, *18*, 369–378. [CrossRef] [PubMed]
5. Naegeli, B.; Kurz, D.J.; Koller, D.; Straumann, E.; Furrer, M.; Maurer, D.; Minder, E.; Bertel, O. Single-chamber ventricular pacing increases markers of left ventricular dysfunction compared with dual-chamber pacing. *Europace* **2007**, *9*, 194–199. [CrossRef] [PubMed]
6. Leclercq, C.; Cazeau, S.; Lellouche, D.; Fossati, F.; Anselme, F.; Davy, J.-M.; Sadoul, N.; Klug, D.; Mollo, L.; Daubert, J.-C. Upgrading from Single Chamber Right Ventricular to Biventricular Pacing in Permanently Paced Patients with Worsening Heart Failure: The RD-CHF Study. *Pacing Clin. Electrophysiol.* **2007**, *30*, S23–S30. [CrossRef]
7. Crevelari, E.S.; Da Silva, K.R.; Albertini, C.M.D.M.; Vieira, M.L.C.; Filho, M.M.; Costa, R. Efficacy, Safety, and Performance of Isolated Left vs. Right Ventricular Pacing in Patients with Bradyarrhythmias: A Randomized Controlled Trial. *Arq. Bras. Cardiol.* **2018**, *112*, 410–421. [CrossRef] [PubMed]
8. Stockburger, M.; de Teresa, E.; Lamas, G.; Desaga, M.; Koenig, C.; Habedank, D.; Cobo, E.; Navarro, X.; Wiegand, U.; Mode Selection Trial (MOST) Investigators. Exercise capacity and N-terminal pro-brain natriuretic peptide levels with biventricular vs. right ventricular pacing for atrioventricular block: Results from the PREVENT-HF German Substudy. *Europace* **2013**, *16*, 63–70. [CrossRef] [PubMed]
9. Shukla, H.H.; Hellkamp, A.S.; James, E.A.; Flaker, G.C.; Lee, K.L.; Sweeney, M.O.; Lamas, G.A. Heart failure hospitalization is more common in pacemaker patients with sinus node dysfunction and a prolonged paced QRS duration. *Heart Rhythm* **2005**, *2*, 245–251. [CrossRef]
10. Connolly, S.J.; Kerr, C.R.; Gent, M.; Roberts, R.S.; Yusuf, S.; Gillis, A.M.; Sami, M.H.; Talajic, M.; Tang, A.S.; Klein, G.J.; et al. Effects of Physiologic Pacing versus Ventricular Pacing on the Risk of Stroke and Death Due to Cardiovascular Causes. Canadian Trial of Physiologic Pacing Investigators. *N. Engl. J. Med.* **2000**, *342*, 1385–1391. [CrossRef]
11. Nielsen, J.C.; Thomsen, P.E.B.; Højberg, S.; Møller, M.; Vesterlund, T.; Dalsgaard, D.; Mortensen, L.S.; Nielsen, T.; Asklund, M.; Friis, E.V.; et al. A comparison of single-lead atrial pacing with dual-chamber pacing in sick sinus syndrome. *Eur. Heart J.* **2011**, *32*, 686–696. [CrossRef] [PubMed]
12. Brignole, M.; Botto, G.; Mont, L.; Iacopino, S.; De Marchi, G.; Oddone, D.; Luzi, M.; Tolosana, J.M.; Navazio, A.; Menozzi, C. Cardiac resynchronization therapy in patients undergoing atrioventricular junction ablation for permanent atrial fibrillation: A randomized trial. *Eur. Heart J.* **2011**, *32*, 2420–2429. [CrossRef] [PubMed]

13. Solomon, S.D.; Foster, E.; Bourgoun, M.; Shah, A.; Viloria, E.; Brown, M.W.; Hall, W.J.; Pfeffer, M.A.; Moss, A.J. Effect of Cardiac Resynchronization Therapy on Reverse Remodeling and Relation to Outcome: Multicenter automatic defibrillator implantation trial: Cardiac resynchronization therapy. *Circulation* **2010**, *122*, 985–992. [CrossRef] [PubMed]
14. Diab, I.G.; Hunter, R.J.; Kamdar, R.; Berriman, T.; Duncan, E.; Richmond, L.; Baker, V.; Abrams, D.; Earley, M.J.; Sporton, S.; et al. Does ventricular dyssynchrony on echocardiography predict response to cardiac resynchronisation therapy? A randomised controlled study. *Heart* **2011**, *97*, 1410–1416. [CrossRef] [PubMed]
15. Young, J.B.; Abraham, W.T.; Smith, A.L.; Leon, A.R.; Lieberman, R.; Wilkoff, B.; Canby, R.C.; Schroeder, J.S.; Liem, L.B.; Hall, S.; et al. Combined Cardiac Resynchronization and Implantable Cardioversion Defibrillation in Advanced Chronic Heart Failure. *JAMA* **2003**, *289*, 2685–2694. [CrossRef]
16. Botto, G.L.; Iuliano, A.; Occhetta, E.; Belotti, G.; Russo, G.; Campari, M.; Valsecchi, S.; Stabile, G. A randomized controlled trial of cardiac resynchronization therapy in patients with prolonged atrioventricular interval: The REAL-CRT pilot study. *Europace* **2019**, *22*, 299–305. [CrossRef]
17. Sweeney, M.O.; Ellenbogen, K.A.; Tang, A.S.; Whellan, D.; Mortensen, P.T.; Giraldi, F.; Sandler, D.A.; Sherfesee, L.; Sheldon, T.; Managed Ventricular Pacing Versus VVI 40 Pacing Trial Investigators. Atrial pacing or ventricular backup–only pacing in implantable cardioverter-defibrillator patients. *Heart Rhythm* **2010**, *7*, 1552–1560. [CrossRef]
18. Abraham, W.T.; Young, J.B.; Leon, A.R.; Adler, S.; Bank, A.J.; Hall, S.A.; Lieberman, R.; Liem, L.B.; O'Connell, J.B.; Schroeder, J.S.; et al. Effects of Cardiac Resynchronization on Disease Progression in Patients With Left Ventricular Systolic Dysfunction, an Indication for an Implantable Cardioverter-Defibrillator, and Mildly Symptomatic Chronic Heart Failure. *Circulation* **2004**, *110*, 2864–2868. [CrossRef]
19. Stockburger, M.; Doblas, J.J.G.; Lamas, G.; Alzueta, J.; Lozano, I.F.; Cobo, E.; Wiegand, U.; De La Concha, J.F.; Navarro, X.; Navarro-López, F.; et al. Preventing ventricular dysfunction in pacemaker patients without advanced heart failure: Results from a multicentre international randomized trial (PREVENT-HF). *Eur. J. Heart Fail.* **2011**, *13*, 633–641. [CrossRef]
20. Orlov, M.V.; Gardin, J.M.; Slawsky, M.; Bess, R.L.; Cohen, G.; Bailey, W.; Plumb, V.; Flathmann, H.; De Metz, K. Biventricular pacing improves cardiac function and prevents further left atrial remodeling in patients with symptomatic atrial fibrillation after atrioventricular node ablation. *Am. Heart J.* **2010**, *159*, 264–270. [CrossRef]
21. Doshi, R.N.; Daoud, E.G.; Fellows, C.; Turk, K.; Duran, A.; Hamdan, M.H.; Pires, L.A.; for the PAVE Study Group. Left Ventricular-Based Cardiac Stimulation Post AV Nodal Ablation Evaluation (The PAVE Study). *J. Cardiovasc. Electrophysiol.* **2005**, *16*, 1160–1165. [CrossRef] [PubMed]
22. Brignole, M.; Menozzi, C.; Gianfranchi, L.; Musso, G.; Mureddu, R.; Bottoni, N.; Lolli, G. Assessment of Atrioventricular Junction Ablation and VVIR Pacemaker versus Pharmacological Treatment in Patients with Heart Failure and Chronic Atrial Fibrillation: A randomized, controlled study. *Circulation* **1998**, *98*, 953–960. [CrossRef] [PubMed]
23. Yu, C.-M.; Lin, H.; Fung, W.-H.; Zhang, Q.; Kong, S.-L.; Sanderson, J.E. Comparison of acute changes in left ventricular volume, systolic and diastolic functions, and intraventricular synchronicity after biventricular and right ventricular pacing for heart failure. *Am. Heart J.* **2003**, *145*, 846. [CrossRef]
24. Yu, C.-M.; Fang, F.; Luo, X.-X.; Zhang, Q.; Azlan, H.; Razali, O. Long-term follow-up results of the Pacing to Avoid Cardiac Enlargement (PACE) trial. *Eur. J. Heart Fail.* **2014**, *16*, 1016–1025. [CrossRef] [PubMed]
25. Sutton, M.S.J.; Plappert, T.; Adamson, P.B.; Li, P.; Christman, S.A.; Chung, E.S.; Curtis, A.B. Left Ventricular Reverse Remodeling with Biventricular versus Right Ventricular Pacing in Patients With Atrioventricular Block and Heart Failure in the BLOCK HF Trial. *Circ. Heart Fail.* **2015**, *8*, 510–518. [CrossRef]
26. Albertsen, A.E.; Nielsen, J.C.; Poulsen, S.H.; Mortensen, P.T.; Pedersen, A.K.; Hansen, P.S.; Jensen, H.K.; Egeblad, H. DDD(R)-pacing, but not AAI(R)-pacing induces left ventricular desynchronization in patients with sick sinus syndrome: Tissue-Doppler and 3D echocardiographic evaluation in a randomized controlled comparison. *Europace* **2008**, *10*, 127–133. [CrossRef]
27. Yu, C.-M.; Chan, J.Y.-S.; Zhang, Q.; Omar, R.; Yip, G.W.-K.; Hussin, A.; Fang, F.; Lam, K.H.; Chan, H.C.-K.; Fung, J.W.-H. Biventricular Pacing in Patients with Bradycardia and Normal Ejection Fraction. *N. Engl. J. Med.* **2009**, *361*, 2123–2134. [CrossRef]
28. Gierula, J.; Cubbon, R.M.; Jamil, H.A.; Byrom, R.; Baxter, P.D.; Pavitt, S.; Gilthorpe, M.S.; Hewison, J.; Kearney, M.T.; Witte, K.K. Cardiac resynchronization therapy in pacemaker-dependent patients with left ventricular dysfunction. *Europace* **2013**, *15*, 1609–1614. [CrossRef]
29. Xu, H.; Xie, X.; Li, J.; Zhang, Y.; Xu, C.; Yang, J. Early Right Ventricular Apical Pacing-Induced Gene Expression Alterations Are Associated with Deterioration of Left Ventricular Systolic Function. *Dis. Markers* **2017**, *2017*, 8405196. [CrossRef] [PubMed]
30. Mitov, V.M.; Perišić, Z.; Jolic, A.; Kostic, T.; Aleksic, A.; Aleksic, Z. The effect of right ventricular pacemaker lead position on functional status in patients with preserved left ventricular ejection fraction. *Med. Rev.* **2016**, *69*, 212–216. [CrossRef]
31. Kaye, G.C.; Linker, N.J.; Marwick, T.H.; Pollock, L.; Graham, L.; Pouliot, E.; Poloniecki, J.; Gammage, M.; Martin, P.; Pepper, C.; et al. Effect of right ventricular pacing lead site on left ventricular function in patients with high-grade atrioventricular block: Results of the Protect-Pace study. *Eur. Heart J.* **2014**, *36*, 856–862. [CrossRef]
32. Molina, L.; Sutton, R.; Gandoy, W.; Reyes, N.; Lara, S.; Limón, F.; Gómez, S.; Orihuela, C.; Salame, L.; Moreno, G. Medium-Term Effects of Septal and Apical Pacing in Pacemaker-Dependent Patients: A Double-Blind Prospective Randomized Study. *Pacing Clin. Electrophysiol.* **2013**, *37*, 207–214. [CrossRef]

33. Lewicka-Nowak, E.; Dabrowska-Kugacka, A.; Tybura, S.; Krzymińska-Stasiuk, E.; Wilczek, R.; Staniewicz, J.; Swiatecka, G.; Raczek, G. Right ventricular apex versus right ventricular outflow tract pacing: Prospective, randomised, long-term clinical and echocardiographic evaluation. *Kardiologia Polska* **2006**, *64*.
34. Zhang, H.X.; Qian, J.; Hou, F.Q.; Liu, Y.N.; Mao, J.H. Comparison of right ventricular apex and right ventricular outflow tract septum pacing in the elderly with normal left ventricular ejection fraction: Long-term follow-up. *Kardiologia Polska* **2012**, *70*, 1130–1139. [PubMed]
35. Flevari, P.; Leftheriotis, D.; Fountoulaki, K.; Panou, F.; Rigopoulos, A.G.; Paraskevaidis, I.; Kremastinos, D.T. Long-Term Nonoutflow Septal Versus Apical Right Ventricular Pacing: Relation to Left Ventricular Dyssynchrony. *Pacing Clin. Electrophysiol.* **2009**, *32*, 354–362. [CrossRef] [PubMed]
36. Gong, X.; Su, Y.; Pan, W.; Cui, J.; Liu, S.; Shu, X. Is Right Ventricular Outflow Tract Pacing Superior to Right Ventricular Apex Pacing in Patients with Normal Cardiac Function? *Clin. Cardiol.* **2009**, *32*, 695–699. [CrossRef] [PubMed]
37. Cano, O.; Osca, J.; Sancho-Tello, M.-J.; Sánchez, J.M.; Ortiz, V.; Castro, J.E.; Salvador, A.; Olagüe, J. Comparison of Effectiveness of Right Ventricular Septal Pacing versus Right Ventricular Apical Pacing. *Am. J. Cardiol.* **2010**, *105*, 1426–1432. [CrossRef] [PubMed]
38. Leong, D.P.; Mitchell, A.-M.; Salna, I.; Brooks, A.G.; Sharma, G.; Lim, H.S.; Alasady, M.; Barlow, M.; Leitch, J.; Sanders, P.; et al. Long-Term Mechanical Consequences of Permanent Right Ventricular Pacing: Effect of Pacing Site. *J. Cardiovasc. Electrophysiol.* **2010**, *21*, 1120–1126. [CrossRef]
39. Nielsen, J.C.; Kristensen, L.; Andersen, H.R.; Mortensen, P.T.; Pedersen, O.L.; Pedersen, A.K. A randomized comparison ofatrial and dual-chamber pacing in177 consecutive patients with sick sinus syndrome: Echocardiographic and clinical outcome. *J. Am. Coll. Cardiol.* **2003**, *42*, 614–623. [CrossRef]
40. Gierula, J.; Jamil, H.A.; Byrom, R.; Joy, E.R.; Cubbon, R.M.; Kearney, M.T.; Witte, K.K. Pacing-associated left ventricular dysfunction? Think reprogramming first! *Heart* **2014**, *100*, 765–769. [CrossRef]
41. Stockburger, M.; Boveda, S.; Moreno, J.; Da Costa, A.; Hatala, R.; Brachmann, J.; Butter, C.; Seara, J.G.; Rolando, M.; Defaye, P. Long-term clinical effects of ventricular pacing reduction with a changeover mode to minimize ventricular pacing in a general pacemaker population. *Eur. Heart J.* **2014**, *36*, 151–157. [CrossRef]
42. Botto, G.L.; Ricci, R.P.; Bénézet, J.M.; Nielsen, J.C.; De Roy, L.; Piot, O.; Quesada, A.; Quaglione, R.; Vaccari, D.; Garutti, C.; et al. Managed ventricular pacing compared with conventional dual-chamber pacing for elective replacement in chronically paced patients: Results of the Prefer for Elective Replacement Managed Ventricular Pacing randomized study. *Heart Rhythm* **2014**, *11*, 992–1000. [CrossRef] [PubMed]
43. Kiehl, E.L.; Makki, T.; Kumar, R.; Gumber, D.; Kwon, D.H.; Rickard, J.W.; Kanj, M.; Wazni, O.M.; Saliba, W.I.; Varma, N.; et al. Incidence and predictors of right ventricular pacing-induced cardiomyopathy in patients with complete atrioventricular block and preserved left ventricular systolic function. *Heart Rhythm* **2016**, *13*, 2272–2278. [CrossRef] [PubMed]
44. Albertsen, A.E.; Nielsen, J.C.; Poulsen, S.H.; Mortensen, P.T.; Pedersen, A.K.; Hansen, P.S.; Jensen, H.K.; Egeblad, H. Biventricular pacing preserves left ventricular performance in patients with high-grade atrio-ventricular block: A randomized comparison with DDD(R) pacing in 50 consecutive patients. *Europace* **2008**, *10*, 314–320. [CrossRef] [PubMed]
45. Weizong, W.; Zhongsu, W.; Yujiao, Z.; Mei, G.; Jiangrong, W.; Yong, Z.; Xinxing, X.; Yinglong, H. Effects of Right Ventricular Nonapical Pacing on Cardiac Function: A Meta-analysis of Randomized Controlled Trials. *Pacing Clin. Electrophysiol.* **2013**, *36*, 1032–1051. [CrossRef] [PubMed]
46. Shimony, A.; Eisenberg, M.J.; Filion, K.; Amit, G. Beneficial effects of right ventricular non-apical vs. apical pacing: A systematic review and meta-analysis of randomized-controlled trials. *Europace* **2011**, *14*, 81–91. [CrossRef]
47. Albakri, A.; Bimmel, D. Right ventricular septal or apical? which is optimal positioning in pacemaker implantation: A systematic review and meta-analysis. *Integr. Mol. Med.* **2020**, *8*, 1–7. [CrossRef]
48. Moss, A.J.; Zareba, W.; Hall, W.J.; Klein, H.; Wilber, D.J.; Cannom, D.S.; Daubert, J.P.; Higgins, S.L.; Brown, M.W.; Andrews, M.L.; et al. Prophylactic implantation of a defibrillator in patients with myocardial infarction and reduced ejection fraction. *N. Engl. J. Med.* **2002**, *346*, 877–883. [CrossRef]
49. Sweeney, M.O.; Hellkamp, A.S. Heart Failure During Cardiac Pacing. *Circulation* **2006**, *113*, 2082–2088. [CrossRef]
50. Muoneme, A.S.; Isiguzo, G.C.; Iroezindu, M.O.; Okeahialam, B.N. Relationship between Six-Minute Walk Test and Left Ventricular Systolic Function in Nigerian Patients with Heart Failure. *West Afr. J. Med.* **2015**, *34*, 133–138.
51. Opasich, C.; Pinna, G.; Capomolla, S.; Mazza, A.; Febo, O.; Riccardi, R.; Forni, G.; Cobelli, F.; Tavazzi, L. Six-minute walking performance in patients with moderate-to-severe heart failure; is it a useful indicator in clinical practice? *Eur. Heart J.* **2001**, *22*, 488–496. [CrossRef] [PubMed]

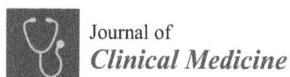

Article

Challenges for Management of Dilated Cardiomyopathy during COVID-19 Pandemic—A Telemedicine Application

Luminita Iliuta [1,2], Andreea Gabriella Andronesi [3,4,*], Eugenia Panaitescu [1], Madalina Elena Rac-Albu [1], Alexandru Scafa-Udriște [5,6] and Horațiu Moldovan [5,7,8]

[1] Medical Informatics and Biostatistics Department, University of Medicine and Pharmacy "Carol Davila", 050474 Bucharest, Romania
[2] Cardioclass Clinic for Cardiovascular Disease, 031125 Bucharest, Romania
[3] Nephrology Department, University of Medicine and Pharmacy "Carol Davila", 050474 Bucharest, Romania
[4] Nephrology Department, Fundeni Clinical Institute, 022328 Bucharest, Romania
[5] Department of Cardio-Thoracic Pathology, University of Medicine and Pharmacy "Carol Davila", 050474 Bucharest, Romania
[6] Department of Cardiology, Clinical Emergency Hospital, 014461, Bucharest, Romania
[7] Department of Cardiovascular Surgery, Clinical Emergency Hospital, 014461 Bucharest, Romania
[8] Academy of Romanian Scientists (AOSR), 3 Ilfov Street, 050044 Bucharest, Romania
* Correspondence: andreea.andronesi@umfcd.ro

Citation: Iliuta, L.; Andronesi, A.G.; Panaitescu, E.; Rac-Albu, M.E.; Scafa-Udriște, A.; Moldovan, H. Challenges for Management of Dilated Cardiomyopathy during COVID-19 Pandemic—A Telemedicine Application. *J. Clin. Med.* **2022**, *11*, 7411. https://doi.org/10.3390/jcm11247411

Academic Editors: Mario J. Garcia and Fatih Yalcin

Received: 24 November 2022
Accepted: 12 December 2022
Published: 14 December 2022

Publisher's Note: MDPI stays neutral with regard to jurisdictional claims in published maps and institutional affiliations.

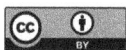

Copyright: © 2022 by the authors. Licensee MDPI, Basel, Switzerland. This article is an open access article distributed under the terms and conditions of the Creative Commons Attribution (CC BY) license (https://creativecommons.org/licenses/by/4.0/).

Abstract: Background and Objectives: The 2019 coronavirus pandemic (COVID-19) represented a significant challenge for the medical community. The first aim of this study was to examine the COVID-19 impact on the follow-up of patients with dilated cardiomyopathy (DCM) and to establish the advantages of multiparametric home monitoring. Also, we tried to establish the main prognostic predictors at 2-years follow-up and the value of LV diastolic filling pattern (LVDFP) in increasing mortality and morbidity. Materials and Methods: We conducted a prospective study of 142 patients with DCM assessed by in-patient visit in the pre-pandemic period and hybrid (face-to-face, online consultation and telemedicine home monitoring with a dedicated application) during the pandemic period. The statistical analysis compared the strategy used in the pre-pandemic with management during the pandemic, in terms of clinical assessment, hospitalizations/emergency room visits due to HF exacerbation and total mortality. Results: We did not observe significant changes in blood pressure (BP), heart rate (FC), weight and symptoms or an increased rate of adverse drug events between the two periods. We successfully titrated HF medications with close monitoring of HF decompensations, which were similar in number, but were mostly managed at home during the pandemic. There was also no statistically significant difference in emergency room visits due to severe decompensated HF. Mortality in the first and second year of follow-up was between 12.0 and 13%, similar in the pre-pandemic and pandemic periods, but significantly higher in patients with restrictive LVDFP. Clinical improvement or stability after 2 years was more frequent in patients with nonrestrictive LVDFP. The main prognostic predictors at 1 and 2-years follow-up were: the restrictive LVDFP, significantly dilated LV, comorbidities (DM, COPD), older age, associated severe mitral regurgitation and pulmonary hypertension. Conclusions: The pandemic restrictions determined a marked decrease of the healthcare use, but no significant change in the clinical status of DCM patients under multiparametric home monitoring. At 2-years follow-up, the presence of the restrictive LVDFP was associated with an increased risk of death and with a worse clinical status in DCM patients.

Keywords: remote monitoring; heart failure; COVID-19; telemedicine; dilated cardiomyopathy; diastolic dysfunction; restrictive pattern

1. Introduction

Dilated cardiomyopathy (DCM) represents a significant cause of morbidity and mortality between patients with heart failure (HF) and aging population. Its evolution is often ondulatory and difficult to predict on short and long-term, especially in patients with multiple comorbidities [1,2]. Despite modern therapy and progresses on surgical treatment, the overall prognostic of this disease remains poor, with a 50% mortality at 5 years [3,4], comparable with that for some of the most frequent neoplasia. Cardiologist is in the position to choose between using different parameters in order to evaluate the severity and the prognosis of the disease and to improve therapeutic management [5].

On the other hand, the global pandemic Coronavirus disease 2019 (COVID-19) impacted significantly the patients' access to telehealth-care system. All specialties were affected by the changes in clinical prioritization, but especially cardiac patients who often need close medical monitoring. In order to reduce viral transmission, many countries introduced lockdown, but these restrictions affected vulnerable patients, like those with HF. Due to advanced age and comorbidities, especially diabetes mellitus (DM), patients with HF have a higher risk of serious infections, including COVID-19, but we have to take into account that, during pandemic, their evaluation also was impacted by reduced social contacts, decreased physical activity and reduced access to healthcare.

In Romania, a state of national emergency was declared from 16 March to 14 May 2020, which implied functioning of only essential services and the advice of staying at home for the general population. The lockdown had a profound impact on the workflow of the hospitals. The entire healthcare system had to reorganize to withstand the pandemic and to find a solution for the care of high-risk patients, such as HF patients. Remote follow-up visits with the use in most cases of phone-calls for stable HF patients were recommended, and the direct patient-doctor contact was reserved for the emergencies.

In recent years, HF management has made important progress, focusing on treatment modalities based not only on traditional drugs, but on various devices to meet the requirements of this complex syndrome. Virtual care models of telemedicine are used to follow-up patients with cardiac implantable electronic devices (CIEDs) and home sensors (wireless pulmonary artery haemodynamic monitoring system) and they have already proved to be efficient in monitoring HF patients in different trials [6–10]. Also, there is increasing interest in expanding virtual CIED care models, including pacemakers, implantable cardioverter defibrillators, and cardiac resynchronization therapy to reduce mortality and hospitalizations in patients with HF. Unfortunately, not all countries benefit from the economic resources necessary for the large-scale application of these devices. In our country, there is a small percentage of patients with HF who benefit from remote monitoring devices, so that, in the context of the pandemic, access to cardiovascular care had to be based on classic remote monitoring. In this context, telemedicine is useful in reducing space and time barriers, thus increasing patients' compliance. However, little is known about the importance of use of the telemedicine in pandemic or lockdown situations.

For this reasons, we aimed to characterize the impact of remote monitoring using a dedicated telemedicine application during the COVID-19 pandemic in our country in patients with DCM and without using interogation of implanted devices. We immediately adapted our clinic dedicated application in order to keep the follow-up of the stable patients with the minimum possible physical contact and we reserved the face-to-face evaluation and interventions for unstable patients. That is why, the first objective of our study was to examine the impact of the COVID-19 pandemic on the healthcare system use and on the clinical status and evolution of patients with DCM under multiparametric home monitoring in a cardiovascular clinic from Bucharest.

On the other hand, a lot of studies revealed that the presence of a restrictive LV diastolic filling pattern (LVDFP) involves a more unfavorable prognosis in most of cardiac diseases (coronary, valvular or congenital) [11–13]. Also, diastolic dysfunction seems to be one of the earliest detectable abnormalities in a lot of the heart disorders. In DCM, the long and medium-term prognosis is influenced by many parameters, amongst which LV diastolic performance is one of the most important [14]. The second purpose of this study was to establish the medium-term prognostic predictors and the implication of the LVDFP on the evolution of patients with DCM at 2-years follow-up.

2. Materials and Methods

2.1. Study Population, Setting, and Data Collection

We carried out a prospective study in 142 patients with DCM evaluated between 1 March 2019 and 1 March 2022. All patients were recorded in the dedicated application of the Cardioclass clinic for cardiovascular disease at least 1 month before the beginning of the national lockdown. Patients were eligible for enrolment if they were diagnosed with DCM and had been evaluated in our clinic and registered in the dedicated application within the previous 12 months. All patients included in this study signed the informed consent form (approved by the institutional ethics committee) in which they authorized the prospective collection of data for research purposes.

In the pre-pandemic period (from 1 March 2019 to 1 March 2020), patients' standard follow-up consisted of in-person appointments (minimum of one appointment per trimester) with a cardiologist physician consultation, ecocardiographic examination and/or ambulatory electrocardiogram or blood pressure monitoring. All patients registered in our clinic had also access to a specific phone number (allocated to nursing staff) to contact the team in case of any warning sign or symptom using a self-monitoring register for vital signs, symptoms and weight. For this home-monitoring we provided before pandemic period for all our HF patients learning instruments, but the data obtained were not included in our dedicated application. We had also a dedicated email for the patients with HF in order to facilitate communication. In some cases, we scheduled follow-up phone calls to better evaluate the patients' symptoms and eventually to adjust treatment, mainly the diuretics doses. Whenever it became necessary, patients with congestion signs and poor response to oral diuretics had been admitted to our clinic in order to administer intravenous diuretics, using a pre-specified protocol.

During the restricted-pandemic period (from 1 March 2020 to 1 March 2021), the face-to-face appointments were reduced drastically (with no visits in the lockdown till 15 May 2020), and there were limited to urgent situations and to patients in NYHA classes III/ambulatory IV (who were however fully evaluated face-to-face, including by echocardiography at least once a year). All appointments scheduled before pandemic period were changed to remote consultations (on-line or phone appointments, including drug prescriptions using email or short message service, with ambulatory adjustments of drugs) and with careful identification of the patients who would need an in-person care. In order to check for drug compliance, we monitored the need for drug prescription renewal. Also, most of the blood tests were performed locally, allowing home-based phlebotomies. More than half of the analysis were obtained directly from the laboratory that processed them. For the rest, the results were sent by email or by phone via WhatsApp to our nurses and entered in the dedicated application. In urgent cases, ambulatory monitoring of electrocardiography (ECG) and blood pressure and transthoracic echocardiograms (with a portable Vivid machine) were performed, but all the stress tests were cancelled.

During pandemic, all patients were home monitored with a multiparametric application (linked with our dedicated software platform) that included daily heart rate (HR), blood pressure (BP), body weight and symptom status. The receiving application could additionally incorporate blood test results and electrocardiograms (via Istel HR-2000 remote monitoring system). This application allows for weekly transmissions of all the monitored parameters and sometimes blood test results and electrocardiograms to the remote monitoring server. Collected data were evaluated and filtered by a specialized team of nurses and physicians in the application and relevant medication changes were communicated to the patients. Also, the monitored parameters were subject to alerts based on pre-specified cut-off absolute values or variations over time.

The main alerts for HF decompensation diagnosis were:

- weight gain more than 4 kg in comparison to the patient's reference weight or weight gain more than 2 kg in five consecutive days;
- mean HR more than 100 b/min in three consecutive days
- increase of blood urea or NT-proBNP more than 30% from the last known value

worsening of HF symptoms based on our dedicated questionnaire.

For simplification of monitoring process and the alerts system, the responses to questions related to HF symptoms were grouped and classified as Good, Attention and Alarm as follows:

Good—No shortness of breath at rest
- Weight gain in one day less than 1–1.5 kg
- No swelling of feet, ankles, legs or belly
- No chest pain
- Non restricted daily activities

Attention—Feel more tired or have worsening shortness of breath at activities or you need more pillows to sleep or you can only sleep while sitting
- Weight gain in one day more than 1–1.5 kg or more than 2.5 kg in one week
- Swelling of feet, ankles, legs or belly
- Dry cough
- You feel more depressed than usual

Alarm—Shortness of breath at rest
- You wake up at night because you cannot breathe
- Weight gain of more than 3.5 kg in one week
- Important swelling of feet, ankles, legs or belly
- You have pain, pressure or tightness in your chest
- You feel confused or dizzy and can't think clearly

Also, through the dedicated application and during the "face-to-face visits", we evaluated two aspects of the global quality of life using a self-reported questionnaire: the physical component (PCS) and the mental component (MCS). The allocated points started from 0 (lowest) up to 10 (highest quality of life). Patients evaluated their change in mental and physical quality of life by answering at the question: "How would you rate your quality of life now?". They had to choose between "Better than previous visit," "The same as previous visit," and "Worse than previous visit".

Visits at the emergency units due to the decompensations of the HF were defined as ambulatory day-admissions, with the administration of intravenous diuretics, while hospitalizations were considered in-hospital admissions for intravenous diuretics or admissions to the intensive care unit for administration of inotropic support.

In the relaxed-pandemic period (from 1 March 2021 to 1 March 2022), we provided a hybrid follow-up of the patients with in-person appointments (minimum of one appointment per year—which included a cardiologist consultation, ecocardiographic examination and/or ambulatory ECG or blood pressure monitoring) and telemedicine consultations (on-line or phone appointments and the use of the dedicated multiparametric application).

Variables of interest were compared between three periods: pre-pandemic (1 March 2019–1 March 2020), restricted-pandemic (1 March 2020, including during lockdown from 16 March to 14th of May 2020 and then till 1 March 2021) and during relaxed-pandemic period from 1 March 2021 to 1 March 2022.

Physiological variables and episodes of decompensations of the HF were evaluated at the enrollment and during the following three years. The telemedicine monitoring application collected data on symptoms, heart rate, weight, blood pressure, ECG, blood tests, HF decompensation episodes, changes in the prescriptions, other medical consultations, and details regarding potential hospitalizations. Moderately HF decompensations resulted in treatment adjustments, including diuretics augmentation.

2.2. Ultrasound Methods

The patients were evaluated by echocardiography at the enrollment (pre-pandemic) and during pandemic, at least one ecocardiographic evaluation every year. We used a Philips Affinity30 or a portable General Electric VIVID machine, with a 3.5 MHz probe for all examinations. All techniques and calculations respected the recommendations of the European and American Society of Echocardiography [14].

At each visit, the main parameters assessed were: dimensions of the heart cavities (left ventricle- LV- end-systolic and end-diastolic diameters and volume, left atrium- LA- diameters, including LA indexed volume) and LV systolic and diastolic performance (with all Tissue Doppler- TDI- parameters measurement) [15].

We used a modified Simpson's method for left ventricular ejection fraction (LVEF) calculation and we record the transmitral flow placing the pulsed wave Doppler (PW) between the mitral leaflet in an apical 4-chamber view. Using PW evaluation, we measured the transmitral flow velocities (Peak Early Diastolic velocity—E wave and late Diastolic velocity—A wave) and the deceleration time (DT). For TDI measurements we placed the PW sample volume in the lateral mitral annulus in the same apical 4-chamber view. We recorded peak annular systolic velocity (Sa), early diastolic velocity (Ea) and late diastolic velocity (Aa).

We classified the LV diastolic performance using LVDFP as follows:
- normal LVDFP (E/A > 1, DT < 220 ms, IVRT = 60–100 ms, Ea/Aa > 1),
- impaired relaxation (E/A < 1, DT > 220 ms, IVRT > 100 ms, Ea/Aa < 1),
- pseudonormalization: (E/A = 1–2, DT = 150–200 ms, IVRT < 100 ms Ea/Aa < 1), and
- restrictive pattern (E/A > 2 or DT < 150 ms, IVRT < 60 ms, Ea/Aa < 1)

Before pandemic period, in order to diagnose the ischemic etiology of DCM, we performed coronary angiography or coronary angio-CT to all patients over 35 years of age, as well as for patients under 35 years old with angina pectoris. 69 patients had associated coronary artery disease (>50% reduction in luminal diameter of any coronary artery). BNP titration was done for all patients at least 3 times per year and for HF diagnosis we consider the age-independent cut-off of 300 pg/mL [16].

All patients were treated with the standard medication for HF including digitalis, diuretics, angiotensin converting enzyme inhibitors and spironolactone. At the moment of enrolment, all the patients were in sinus rhythm.

Depending on the LV systolic function the patients were divided in two groups:

(a) Group A—105 patients with a moderate LV systolic dysfunction (LVEF = 25–35%), and

(b) Group B—37 patients with a severe LV systolic dysfunction (LVEF ≤ 25%).

Depending on both systolic and diastolic function of the LV, each group was divided in two subgroups:
- Subgroup A1—76 patients with a nonrestrictive LVDFP
- Subgroup A2—29 patients with a restrictive LVDFP
- Subgroup B1—19 patients with a non-restrictive LV filling pattern, and
- Subgroup B2—18 patients with a restrictive LV filling pattern (Figure 1).

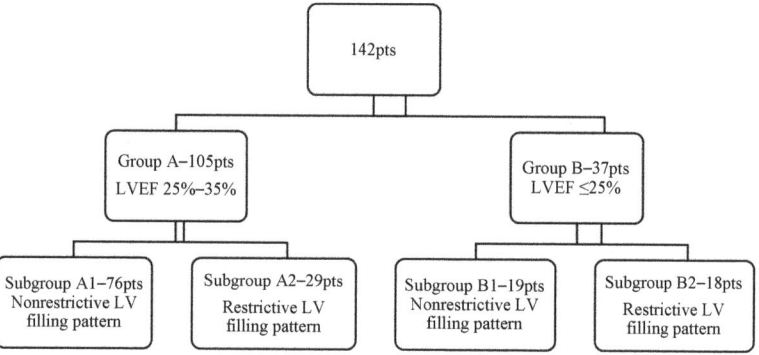

Figure 1. Study group structure depending on LV systolic and diastolic performance.

The demographic characteristics (mean age, gender), secondary mitral regurgitation degree and the mean pulmonary artery pressure were similar in the two study groups.

2.3. Statistical Analysis

We performed statistical analysis using Statistical Package for the Social Sciences, version 18.0 for the regression analysis and calculation of correlation coefficient and relative risk.

Categorical variables are expressed as absolute numbers (percentages). Normally distributed continuous variables are presented as mean ± standard deviation. Non-normal distributions are presented as median (interquartile range). The univariate comparison of baseline characteristics seen before pandemia and those seen during pandemia was made using the chi-squared test, Fisher exact test, Student's *t*-test, or the Kruskal–Wallis test where appropriate. *p* value of <0.05 was considered statistically significant. Taking into account the exploratory nature of the study, for multiple comparisons adjustments were not made.

Categorical variables were tested with the χ2 test. To evaluate the homogeneity of variances Levene's test was used. For testing the differences in mean values of continuous variables we used analysis of variance (ANOVA) with Games-Howell post hoc test for nonequal variances and Tukey post hoc test for equal variances. Wilcoxon test and Friedman test compared pre-pandemic and intra-pandemic variables. The association between pre-pandemic variables and the intra-pandemic change in hospitalizations and quality of life was based on Pearson correlation analysis, and logistic regression analysis established the association between pre-pandemic clinical and ecographical data and mortality or the magnitude of HF severity variation.

For the estimation of the medium-term prognosis the main endpoints used were: type of LVDFP, NYHA class for HF, quality of life and death.

3. Results

Demographic and Clinical Characteristics of the Patients

A total of 144 patients with DCM were eligible for the study; we excluded two patients because of missing data for the period of interest.

Information regarding the demographic, clinical, ecographic characteristics and HF therapies of the patients were obtained before the pandemic period, in the last appointment and is presented in Table 1. The majority of patients received target doses of HF medication in accordance with the current guidelines.

During the restrictive-pandemic period (2020–2021), there were only two patients diagnosed with COVID-19 who were infected in the hospital, with a mild form and favorable outcome (no cardiovascular or respiratory complications, with only mild symptoms). In the second year of follow-up, the percent of the vaccinated patients was more than 90%, and only 24 patients had a mild form of COVID-19.

In the pre-pandemic period, we registered a mean of 10 phone calls per month with a dedicated nurse for HF patients vs. a mean of 25 calls per month during the pandemic. Regarding clinical evaluation, in the pre-pandemic period all of the appointments were in clinic, with heart ultrasound evaluation during each visit. During the pandemic period, more than 80% of all the appointments were done remotely. During the second year of the pandemic period (relaxed-pandemic between March 2021 and March 2022), the number of the patients with in-clinic visits significantly increased compared to March 2020–2021 (restricted-pandemic)—78.17% vs. 19.71%, $p < 0.05$.

Table 1. Baseline clinical and demographic characteristics of the patients n = 142.

	Group A—105 pts LVEF = 25–35%	Group B—37 pts LVEF ≤ 25%	p Value
Mean (SD) age (years)	58 (12)	61 (11)	0.381 [1]
Women	41 (39.05%)	15 (40.54%)	0.584 [2]
Medical history, no. (%)			
Arterial hypertension	49 (46.66%)	18 (48.65%)	0.229 [2]
Diabetes mellitus	55 (52.38%)	20 (54.05%)	0.135 [2]
Paroxistic atrial fibrillation	42 (40%)	16 (43.24%)	0.065 [2]
Ischaemic aetiology of DCM, no. (%)	50 (47.62%)	19 (45.35%)	0.059 [2]
Chronic kidney disease	35 (33.34%)	12 (32.43%)	0.338 [2]
COPD	18 (17.14%)	7 (18.92%)	0.126 [2]
Mean (SD) LVEF (%)	35 (5)	26 (4)	0.03 [1]
Restrictive LVDFP	29 (27.62%)	18 (48.65%)	0.01 [2]
Mean (SD) heart rate	75 (17)	74 (17)	0.64 [1]
Systolic blood pressure (mm Hg)	125 ± 18	111 ± 12	0.052 [1]
NYHA[a] class I/II	40 (38.09%)	5 (13.51%)	
NYHA[a] class III	52 (49.52%)	12 (32.43%)	0.001 [3]
NYHA[a] class IV	13 (12.638%)	20 (54.05%)	
Median NT-proBNP (IQR) [b] (pg/mL)	1192 (800–2693)	1929 (800–2693)	0.034 [1]
Medications, no. (%)			
ACEi or ARB	67 (63.81%)	22 (59.46%)	0.114 [3]
Sacubitril/valsartan	35 (33.34%)	11 (29.73%)	0.212 [3]
Beta-blocker	98 (93.34%)	30 (81.08%)	0.071 [3]
Mineralocorticoid receptor antagonist	99 (94.28%)	35 (94.59%)	0.511 [3]
Ivabradine	10 (9.52%)	3 (8.11%)	0.442 [3]
Digitalis	52 (49.52%)	29 (78.38%)	0.001 [3]
Diuretic	53 (50.48%)	37 (100%)	0.001 [3]
Implantable cardioverter-defibrillator	2 (1.90%)	3 (8.11%)	0.001 [3]

LVEF—left ventricle ejection fraction; LV—left ventricle; NYHA—New York Heart Association; ACEi—angiotensin-converting enzyme inhibitor; ARB—angiotensin receptor blocker; COPD—chronic obstructive pulmonary disease. [a] New York Heart Association (NYHA) class reflects patients' status in the last face-to-face prepandemic appointment. Plus-minus values are means ± standard deviation. [1] ANOVA; [2] Pearson chi-square; [3] Likelihood ratio. [b] NT-pro-BNP denotes N-terminal pro-B-type natriuretic peptide plasma levels expressed as pg/mL and IQR represents interquartile range.

We found that, despite the health care delivery barriers created by the COVID-19 pandemic, the use of telemedicine allowed us to not only continue monitoring patients with DCM, but also to expand the ambulatory treatment of HF decompensations and the cardiovascular counseling and treatment titration.

Even by remote appointments we were able to successfully titrate HF treatment, such as sacubitril/valsartan, with a careful monitoring of ambulatory blood tests results (serum creatinine, potassium and sodium levels), blood pressure, heart rate, weight and symptoms entered by the patients in the dedicated HF platform. There were no significant changes in weight, BP or HR between the study periods and no sustained ventricular arrhythmia occurred during any of the study periods.

The restricted and relaxed pandemic periods were not associated with significant changes in monitored parameters, including medium weight gain/month (1.2 ± 0.562 kg in pre-pandemic period versus 1.13 ± 0.657 kg during pandemic), systolic BP (121 ± 19 mmHg before pandemic versus 121 ± 18 during pandemic), HR (68 ± 10 b/min before pandemic versus 67 ± 10 b/min during pandemic, $p = 0.05$). Also, we did not observe an increased rate of adverse drug events during the online follow-up.

Regarding the self-reported patients' quality of life score, there were no differences regarding the physical component (PCS) before and during pandemic. The mental component (MCS) of the self-reported quality of life was different in the three study periods.

The percent of the patients with a favorable evolution quantified as a self-reported MCS more than five was significantly smaller during the restrictive pandemic period compared with pre-pandemic (80.28% vs. 24.65%) and increased during the relaxed-pandemic period (54.93%, $p < 0.05$).

The number of alerts before and during pandemic were similar. Overall, the remote monitoring center received a similar number of alerts during pandemic than before it, although the numbers of telephone calls were significantly higher during pandemic (3.6 ± 4.1 per patient before pandemic vs. 7.9 ± 3.2 during restricted-pandemic period and 4.6 ± 2.8 during relaxed-pandemic, $p < 0.05$). Blood tests were significantly reduced during the restricted pandemic and especially during the lockdown due to the important decrease in the laboratory visits.

Before pandemic period, 31 patients reported HF decompensations and 29 of them required hospitalization. During restricted pandemic we observed 29 decompensated HF, but 21 pts were managed remotely by online consultation and 6 pts were admitted to our clinic in order to administer intravenous diuretics, using a pre-specified protocol. Most of the patients reported inability to access hospital. Also, more than 80% of the patients stated they would only attend hospital if there was no alternative. During relaxed pandemic there were 32 patients with decompensated HF from which 19 pts were managed online, 8 pts were treated to our clinic with intravenous diuretics and 5 pts needed hospitalisation.

Regarding emergency department visits due to significant HF decompensation, there was no statistically significant difference between the pre-pandemic and the pandemic period ($p = 0.83$).

The global mortality after the first year and second year of follow-up of this cohort (irrespective of the type of the LVDFP) was 11.97%, and 12.8% respectively, which was not significantly different compared to the mortality predicted by the Meta-Analysis Global Group in Chronic Heart Failure risk score at 1 year (mean value of 12.0% + 6.9%) [15]. Also, the number of deaths did not differ significantly in the pre-pandemic period compared to the pandemic.

Taking into account the type of the LVDFP, the mortality at one and 2-years follow-up was significantly higher in the restrictive LVDFP group (17.5% vs. 10.59% in the non-restrictive group for the first year of follow-up, $p < 0.05$, respectively 21.21% in restrictive group vs. 9.21% in the non-restrictive group for the second year of follow-up, $p < 0.05$), regardless of the LV systolic performance.

The presence of the restrictive LVDFP significantly increased the risk of death at 1 year and at 2-year follow up, irrespective of the presence of different parameters recognized to increase mortality in DCM patients. Regression analysis confirmed that the restrictive LVDFP was an independent predictor for increasing the risk of death or hospitalization for HF decompensations ($p = 0.001$), regardless of the LV dimensions or performance, the presence of a hemodynamically significant secondary MR or pulmonary hypertension. Furthermore, the prognosis of the patients with the restrictive pattern was worst, no matter of the other factors involved.

At 2-years follow-up in DCM patients the main parameters associated with unfavorable evolution revealed by multivariate logistic regression analysis were: patient's age more than 75 years (RR = 9.3, $p < 0.01$), significantly dilated LV (end-systolic volume >95 cm3- RR = 6.7, $p < 0.0001$, end-systolic diameter > 55 mm—RR = 6.9, $p < 0.05$), restrictive LVDFP (RR = 10.9, $p < 0.002$), severe MR (RR = 9.8, $p < 0.05$) and severe pulmonary hypertension (RR = 7.8, $p = 0.005$) (Figure 2).

MR- mitral regurgitation; LVESV- left ventricle end-systolic volume; LVEDD- left ventricle end-diastolic diameter; LVEDV- left ventricle end diastolic volume; LVESV- left ventricle end systolic volume PAP- pulmonary arterial pressure

Regarding the patients' clinical course, the percentages of those with a favorable evolution quantified as NYHA class of HF less than 3 and self-reported quality of life score more than five at one- and two-years follow-up were higher in the nonrestrictive LVDFP group. At 1-year follow-up, the percentage of patients with a better or the same quality-of-life score was significantly higher in nonrestrictive LVDFP subgroup of patients compared with the restrictive one (58.13% vs. 13.04%, $p < 0.005$, likelihood ratio). Also, at 1-year follow-up, the percentage of patients in NYHA class less than 3 was four-fold in patients with nonrestrictive LVDFP (42.1% in nonrestrictive LVDFP group vs. 10.52% in restrictive LVDFP group, $p < 0.05$).

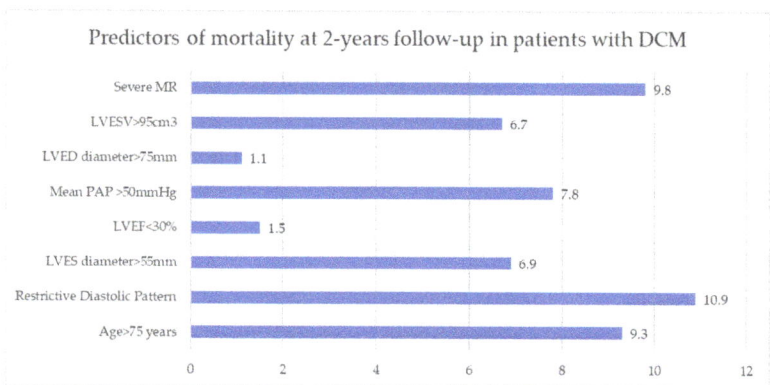

Figure 2. Predictors of mortality at 2-years follow-up in patients with DCM. MR—mitral regurgitation; LVESV—left ventricle end-systolic volume; LVEDD—left ventricle end-diastolic diameter; LVEDV—left ventricle end diastolic volume; LVESV—left ventricle end systolic volume PAP—pulmonary arterial pressure.

4. Discussion

The COVID-19 pandemic has posed a significant challenge to health systems in a multitude of ways. Patients with stable HF no longer had access to hospitals, these being reserved for seriously ill patients in emergency rooms and intensive care units. All clinics have had to adapt and pay attention to stable homebound patients and establish new remote strategies to continue providing quality care.

We found that despite the health-care delivery barriers due to COVID-19, telemedicine allowed us to continue seeing patients with DCM. This is the first study analyzing the impact of telemedicine on cardiovascular management during the COVID-19 pandemic in Romania. Our results support the ongoing use of telemedicine as a means to improve patient access to cardiovascular counseling and testing services.

Due to reduced healthcare contact and lifestyle changes, lockdowns could have a negative impact on HF patient. Our study suggest that our national lockdown had small impact on short-term in our HF patients who were adherent to remote monitoring. In countries with largely developed implanted electronic devices for HF patients (CIED), telemonitoring showed a significant and large reduction in hospitalisation, patients being managed with a wireless implantable haemodynamic monitoring system [17,18].

The TIM-HF2 (Telemedical Interventional Monitoring in Heart Failure) randomized trial proved that remote multiparametric management of patients with HF could reduce unplanned hospitalization rate and death [19]. On the other hand, BEAT-HF (The Better Effectiveness After Transition-Heart Failure) randomized clinical trial demonstrates that remote monitoring after discharge of hospitalized patients with HF using combined health coaching telephone calls and telemonitoring did not reduce 180-day readmissions [20].

We found a positive impact of our telemedicine model on the quality of life and the morbidity and mortality of DCM patients. We compared the data before and during the pandemic, in order to evaluate the impact of our telemedicine application.

The COVID-19 pandemic determined significant anxiety amongst HF patients regarding cancellation of scheduled appointments, investigations, procedures, prescription, and monitoring services. Also, amplifying messages that those with chronic conditions should stay at home and avoid all physical contact may confuse and frighten HF patients, which may result in late presentation to the doctor in case of congestive symptoms. Even worse, patients with severe symptoms, whether due to COVID-19 or the underlying disease, may choose to stay at home with their family rather than risk isolation in the hospital.

During the pandemic, we intensified the number of remote visits and we were able to manage most of them without the need of hospitalization. There was no rise in emergency department visits and hospitalizations due to HF decompensation and no increase in mortality of all-cause, showing that this solution was safe and effective, and permitted also protection against SARS-CoV-2 infection. Due to the increase in telemedical management of HF patients, we were able to maintain a low rate of hospitalizations due to HF decompensation without an increase in mortality. In light of these results, we encourage the progressive use of telemedicine in patients with HF in a pandemic context, but also in situations where physical consultation is difficult for logistical reasons.

On the other hand, when we look at the study design, the first impression is that the HF patients received a lot more attention when they were assessed by telemedicine manners (weekly) compared to the face-to-face consultations (every three months). Although during the prepandemic period we monitored patients at least 1 visit per trimester, all patients registered in our clinic used a self-monitoring register for vital signs, symptoms and weight and had also access to a specific phone number and to a dedicated email (allocated to nursing staff) to contact the team in case of any warning sign or symptom. For this home-monitoring we provided before pandemic period for all our HF patients learning instruments, but the data obtained were not included before pandemic in our dedicated application. Also, even pre-pandemic, in some cases, we scheduled follow-up phone calls to better evaluate the patients' symptoms and to adjust medication. Even so, since all these interventions were not clearly and timely quantified in the dedicated application, the question remains whether the positive results are not mainly because of the telemedicine pros, but because of the more detailed and frequent monitoring of the patients. We hope that, with the improved telemedicine application, in future studies we will be able to clearly clarify this question.

Anyway, with all the problems that the pandemic has involved, COVID-19 has highlighted unprecedented opportunities to expand telemedicine applications for monitoring patients at home. The development of interoperable telemedicine systems would also reduce geographical barriers, which are sometimes very important in the follow-up of patients with DCM. In addition, the time savings achieved through remote consultation offer flexibility to patients and may increase participation for those who are medically or socially vulnerable, or those who do not have immediate access to medical services.

The impact of telemedicine on doctors' practices has been addressed in few previous studies. Positives noted included that telecommuting increased scheduling flexibility and physician availability to patients through online appointments. The negative aspects from the clinician's point of view are related to the lack of face-to-face contact which, in certain situations is essential, and technological limitations. We also faced this in the study, where it was difficult to collaborate with rural or elderly patients.

Thus, to ensure that the delivery of telehealth care meets the needs of both patients and physicians, it is necessary to pay close attention to both technological barriers and human relationship needs. We believe that, by addressing these issues, the implementation of safe and effective virtual care on a large scale for patients with HF will be facilitated [21].

Our study reinforces what other studies have found. It is important to create telemedicine applications where patients are proactively enrolled and equipped with physiological monitors that can communicate vital information. Applications should include specific questions regarding symptomatology, quality of life, psychological health, physical activity and parameters specific to the chronic condition followed, all of which ensure the correct monitoring of patients and the prompt establishment of the indication for requesting a face-to-face evaluation.

On the other hand, data from the present study are in line with the results from other studies demonstrating that LV diastolic filling is an important predictor of severity and prognosis in DCM [22,23]. The restrictive LVDFP is frequently observed in DCM, especially in most severe forms of the disease, and is the best predictor for cardiac death [24–27]. Thus, in our study, the mortality rate at 2-year follow-up was significantly higher in patients with DCM with restrictive LVDFP compared with those with a nonrestrictive filling pattern. Evaluation by NYHA class and quality of life has shown that improvement at 2-years follow up was more frequent in patients with nonrestrictive LVDFP, same results being obtained in other studies [28–32].

The survival rate at 2-years was 94% in patients with a nonrestrictive filling pattern (defined as prolonged DT) compared to 52% for patients with restrictive LV diastolic filling [23]. The survival rate was 84%, 73% and 61% at 1, 2 and 4 years respectively in another study dealing with DCM patients, that is significantly lower compared to that of age- and gender-matched population. [26]. At the 2-years follow-up, in the group with standard treatment, we found a mortality rate slightly higher than those from the literature, probably because of the transplantation surgery which is not well developed in our country, and also because of the underuse of novel treatments, such as sacubitril.

The risk of death at 2-years follow-up was increased by the important enlargement of the LV, severe MR and severe pulmonary hypertension, as was showed in other previous studies [4,24,27,33–35].

We observed that, in spite of survival of patients with restrictive LVDFP, their quality of life was much worse compared to those with a non-restrictive pattern. Thus, severe systolic dysfunction of the LV has a less influence upon evolution compared to the restrictive LVDFP.

Study Limitations

There are some limitations of our study: it is a single-center observational study, with a small sample size, a medium follow-up period, and a low number of events.

Our study highlighted some of the limitations of telemedicine. 10% of patients failed to go to the testing laboratory, compared with in-person patient appointment when obtaining a patient blood sample was easier. Also, several older patients preferred in-person visits, despite their higher risk for COVID-19, probably due to a lower comfort level with telemedicine technology in older adults. We were unable to perform physical examinations via telemedicine. Also, because of the interoperability problems encountered in our country with patients' medical records, the electronic registries were not systematized and there is no software that may generate an alert email every time one of the DCM patients is admitted to the hospital.

We acknowledge that our results are based on experience gained during a health system crisis and do not represent the general experience in the practice of telemedicine. In our study we did not address the aspects of patient or doctor satisfaction with the dedicated telemedicine application developed in our clinic. Further studies could explore the prospects of expanding this application and the implications of the use of telemedicine over a longer period and not in pandemic crisis conditions both from the perspective of the doctor and the patient. In addition, at the time of designing the application, in full lockdown, we had no information available regarding the specific technical difficulties that might have arisen during remote visits.

Moreover, telemedicine may pose a significant ethical issue regarding protection of personal data, since it is possible that safety breaches may allow, at least in theory, external access to the database [36]. That is why, for the large-scale development of this dedicated telemedicine application, despite its effectiveness, it will have to answer all questions regarding ethical considerations (security and confidentiality of transmitted data, confidentiality and privacy of the patient-doctor relationship).

5. Conclusions

Despite a significant decrease in conventional measures of healthcare use, the clinical status of DCM patients under multiparametric monitoring was affected minimally by pandemic restrictions. This telemedicine strategy, combined with patient education, may reduce significantly and even cancel the health risks associated with strict lockdowns, as well as geographic barriers. The remote monitoring allowed early identification and home management of most of the HF decompensations during pandemic. Our findings suggest that a combination of home remote monitoring with in-patient visits represent a very good tool for preserving the care and safety of patients with DCM.

In patients with DCM, the presence of a restrictive LVDFP is associated with a more unfavorable prognosis, this type of filling increasing the risk of death. Also, restrictive filling involves a worsened clinical status of the patients (quantified as NYHA class and the quality of life).

At 2-years follow-up, the presence of a restrictive LVDFP, second-degree MR, dilated LV with LVESD >55 mm and LVESV > 95 mm^3, and severe pulmonary hypertension can anticipate higher mortality rates in DCM patients.

Author Contributions: Conceptualization, L.I. and A.G.A.; data curation, L.I.; formal analysis, L.I., M.E.R.-A. and A.G.A.; investigation, A.G.A.; methodology, L.I. and A.S.-U.; project administration, L.I.; software, L.I. and E.P.; supervision, L.I.; validation, L.I. and A.G.A.; writing—original draft preparation, L.I., A.S.-U. and A.G.A.; writing—review and editing, A.G.A. and H.M.; All authors have read and agreed to the published version of the manuscript.

Funding: This research received no external funding.

Institutional Review Board Statement: The study was conducted in accordance with the Declaration of Helsinki, and approved by the Institutional Review Board of Cardioclass (protocol code 305 from 7 January 2019).

Informed Consent Statement: Informed consent was obtained from all subjects involved in the study. Written informed consent has been obtained from the patients to publish this paper.

Data Availability Statement: All data generated or analyzed during this study are included in this published article.

Conflicts of Interest: The authors declare no conflict of interest.

Abbreviations

LVDFP—left ventricle diastolic filling pattern; DCM—dilated cardiomyopathy, LV—left ventricle, LVEF—left ventricle ejection fraction, DT—deceleration time, NYHA—New York Heart Association; ED—emergency department; DM—diabetes mellitus; COPD—chronic obstructive pulmonary disease; MR—mitral regurgitation; COVID 19—Coronavirus disease 2019; HR—heart rate; BP—blood pressure; HF—heart failure; ACEi—angiotensin-converting enzyme inhibitor; ARB—angiotensin receptor blocker; LVES—left ventricle end-systolic; LVEDD—left ventricle end-diastolic diameter; LVEDV—left ventricle end diastolic volume; PAP—pulmonary arterial pressure; EDt—E-wave deceleration time; IVRT—isovolumetric relaxation time; TDI—tissue doppler imaging.

References

1. Truby, L.K.; Rogers, J.G. Advanced Heart Failure: Epidemiology, Diagnosis, and Therapeutic Approaches. *JACC Heart Fail.* **2020**, *8*, 523–536. [CrossRef] [PubMed]
2. Schultheiss, H.P.; Fairweather, D.; Caforio, A.L.P.; Escher, F.; Hershberger, R.E.; Lipshultz, S.E.; Liu, P.P.; Matsumori, A.; Mazzanti, A.; McMurray, J.; et al. Dilated cardiomyopathy. *Nat. Rev. Dis. Prim.* **2019**, *5*, 32. [CrossRef]
3. Japp, A.G.; Gulati, A.; Cook, S.A.; Cowie, M.R.; Prasad, S.K. The Diagnosis and Evaluation of Dilated Cardiomyopathy. *J. Am. Coll. Cardiol* **2016**, *67*, 2996–3010. [CrossRef]
4. Macarie, C.; Iliuta, L.; Savulescu, C.; Moldovan, H.; Vasile, R.; Filipescu, D.; Gherghiceanu, D.P.; Candea, V. The left ventricular diastolic filling pattern as prognostic predictor in patients with idiopathic dilated cardiomyopathy. *Eur. Heart J.* **2004**, *25*, 7.

5. Thomas, D.E.; Wheeler, R.; Yousef, Z.R.; Masani, N.D. The role of echocardiography in guiding management in dilated cardiomyopathy. *Eur. J. Echocardiogr.* **2009**, *10*, 15–21. [CrossRef]
6. Afonso Nogueira, M.; Ferreira, F.; Raposo, A.F.; Mónica, L.; Simões Dias, S.; Vasconcellos, R.; Proença, G. Impact of telemedicine on the management of heart failure patients during coronavirus disease 2019 pandemic. *ESC Heart Fail.* **2021**, *8*, 1150–1155. [CrossRef]
7. Ahmed, F.Z.; Blomström-Lundqvist, C.; Bloom, H.; Cooper, C.; Ellis, C.; Goette, A.; Greenspon, A.J.; Love, C.J.; Johansen, J.B.; Philippon, F.; et al. Use of healthcare claims to validate the Prevention of Arrhythmia Device Infection Trial cardiac implantable electronic device infection risk score. *Europace* **2021**, *23*, 1446–1455. [CrossRef]
8. Sankaranarayanan, R.; Hartshorne-Evans, N.; Redmond-Lyon, S.; Wilson, J.; Essa, H.; Gray, A.; Clayton, L.; Barton, C.; Ahmed, F.Z.; Cunnington, C.; et al. The impact of COVID-19 on the management of heart failure: A United Kingdom patient questionnaire study. *ESC Heart Fail.* **2021**, *8*, 1324–1332. [CrossRef]
9. Abraham, W.T.; Adamson, P.B.; Bourge, R.C.; Aaron, M.F.; Costanzo, M.R.; Stevenson, L.W.; Strickland, W.; Neelagaru, S.; Raval, N.; Krueger, S.; et al. Wireless pulmonary artery haemodynamic monitoring in chronic heart failure: A randomised controlled trial. *Lancet* **2011**, *377*, 658–666. [CrossRef]
10. Visco, V.; Esposito, C.; Manzo, M.; Fiorentino, A.; Galasso, G.; Vecchione, C.; Ciccarelli, M. A Multistep Approach to Deal With Advanced Heart Failure: A Case Report on the Positive Effect of Cardiac Contractility Modulation Therapy on Pulmonary Pressure Measured by CardioMEMS. *Front. Cardiovasc. Med.* **2022**, *9*, 874433.
11. Iliuta, L.; Rac-Albu, M. Predictors and late incidence of persistent or recurrent heart failure after aortic valve replacement for aortic stenosis compared with aortic regurgitation. *Eur. Heart J.* **2014**, *35*, 358.
12. Jurcut, R.; Savu, O.; Popescu, B.A.; Florian, A.; Herlea, V.; Moldovan, H.; Ginghina, C. Primary cardiac leiomyosarcoma when valvular disease becomes a vascular surgical emergency. *Circulation* **2010**, *121*, E415–E418. [CrossRef]
13. Iliuta, L. The role of TDI diastolic measurements for prognostic prediction early and late after surgical ventricular reconstruction. *Eur. Heart J.* **2019**, *40*, 2798.
14. Nagueh, S.F.; Smiseth, O.A.; Appleton, C.P.; Byrd, B.F., 3rd; Dokainish, H.; Edvardsen, T.; Flachskampf, F.A.; Gillebert, T.C.; Klein, A.L.; Lancellotti, P.; et al. Recommendations for the Evaluation of Left Ventricular Diastolic Function by Echocardiography: An Update from the American Society of Echocardiography and the European Association of Cardiovascular Imaging. *J. Am. Soc. Echocardiogr.* **2016**, *29*, 277–314. [CrossRef]
15. Henein, M.Y.; Lindqvist, P. Diastolic function assessment by echocardiography: A practical manual for clinical use and future applications. *Echocardiography* **2020**, *37*, 1908–1918. [CrossRef]
16. Januzzi, J.L.; van Kimmenade, R.; Lainchbury, J.; Bayes-Genis, A.; Ordonez-Llanos, J.; Santalo-Bel, M.; Pinto, Y.M.; Richards, M. NT-proBNP testing for diagnosis and short-term prognosis in acute destabilized heart failure: An international pooled analysis of 1256 patients: The International Collaborative of NT-proBNP Study. *Eur. Heart J.* **2006**, *27*, 330–337. [CrossRef]
17. Rich, J.D.; Burns, J.; Freed, B.H.; Maurer, M.S.; Burkhoff, D.; Shah, S.J. Meta-Analysis Global Group in Chronic (MAGGIC) Heart Failure Risk Score: Validation of a Simple Tool for the Prediction of Morbidity and Mortality in Heart Failure With Preserved Ejection Fraction. *J. Am. Heart Assoc.* **2018**, *7*, e009594. [CrossRef]
18. Boehmer, J.P.; Hariharan, R.; Devecchi, F.G.; Smith, A.L.; Molon, G.; Capucci, A.; An, Q.; Averina, V.; Stolen, C.M.; Thakur, P.H.; et al. A Multisensor Algorithm Predicts Heart Failure Events in Patients With Implanted Devices: Results From the MultiSENSE Study. *JACC Heart Fail.* **2017**, *5*, 216–225. [CrossRef]
19. Koehler, F.; Winkler, S.; Schieber, M.; Sechtem, U.; Stangl, K.; Böhm, M.; Boll, H.; Kim, S.S.; Koehler, K.; Lücke, S.; et al. Telemedical Interventional Monitoring in Heart Failure (TIM-HF), a randomized, controlled intervention trial investigating the impact of telemedicine on mortality in ambulatory patients with heart failure: Study design. *Eur. J. Heart Fail.* **2010**, *12*, 1354–1362. [CrossRef]
20. Ong, M.K.; Romano, P.S.; Edgington, S.; Aronow, H.U.; Auerbach, A.D.; Black, J.T.; De Marco, T.; Escarce, J.J.; Evangelista, L.S.; Hanna, B.; et al. Effectiveness of Remote Patient Monitoring After Discharge of Hospitalized Patients With Heart Failure: The Better Effectiveness After Transition—Heart Failure (BEAT-HF) Randomized Clinical Trial. *JAMA Intern. Med.* **2016**, *176*, 310–318. [CrossRef]
21. Breton, M.; Sullivan, E.E.; Deville-Stoetzel, N.; McKinstry, D.; DePuccio, M.; Sriharan, A.; Deslauriers, V.; Dong, A.; McAlearney, A.S. Telehealth challenges during COVID-19 as reported by primary healthcare physicians in Quebec and Massachusetts. *BMC Fam. Pract* **2021**, *22*, 192. [CrossRef] [PubMed]
22. Iliuta, L.; Savulescu, C.; Moldovan, H.; Gherghiceanu, D.P.; Vasile, R.; Filipescu, D. Diastolic versus systolic left ventricular dysfunction as independent predictors for unfavourable postoperative evolution in patients with aortic stenosis undergoing aortic valve replacement. *Eur. Heart J.* **2005**, *26*, 193.
23. Brown, P.F.; Miller, C.; Di Marco, A.; Schmitt, M. Towards cardiac MRI based risk stratification in idiopathic dilated cardiomyopathy. *Heart* **2019**, *105*, 270–275. [CrossRef] [PubMed]
24. Matsumura, Y.; Takata, J.; Kitaoka, H.; Kubo, T.; Baba, Y.; Hoshikawa, E.; Hamada, T.; Okawa, M.; Hitomi, N.; Sato, K.; et al. Long-term prognosis of dilated cardiomyopathy revisited: An improvement in survival over the past 20 years. *Circ. J.* **2006**, *70*, 376–383. [CrossRef] [PubMed]
25. Goldberger, J.J.; Subačius, H.; Patel, T.; Cunnane, R.; Kadish, A.H. Sudden cardiac death risk stratification in patients with nonischemic dilated cardiomyopathy. *J. Am. Coll. Cardiol.* **2014**, *63*, 1879–1889. [CrossRef]

26. Iliuta, L.; Andronesi, A.G.; Diaconu, C.C.; Panaitescu, E.; Camburu, G. Additional Prognostic Value of Tissue Doppler Evaluation in Patients with Aortic Stenosis and Left-Ventricular Systolic Dysfunction Undergoing Aortic Valve Replacement. *Medicina* **2022**, *58*, 1410. [CrossRef]
27. Markman, T.M.; Nazarian, S. Moving Toward Improved Risk Stratification in Patients With Dilated Cardiomyopathy. *Circ. Cardiovasc. Imaging* **2020**, *13*, e010629. [CrossRef]
28. Marrow, B.A.; Cook, S.A.; Prasad, S.K.; McCann, G.P. Emerging Techniques for Risk Stratification in Nonischemic Dilated Cardiomyopathy: JACC Review Topic of the Week. *J. Am. Coll. Cardiol.* **2020**, *75*, 1196–1207. [CrossRef]
29. Anghel, L.; Sascău, R.; Zota, I.M.; Stătescu, C. Well-Known and Novel Serum Biomarkers for Risk Stratification of Patients with Non-ischemic Dilated Cardiomyopathy. *Int. J. Mol. Sci* **2021**, *22*, 5688. [CrossRef]
30. Iliuta, L.; Moldovan, H.; Filipescu, D.; Radulescu, B.; Vasilescu, A. Diastolic versus systolic left ventricular dysfunction as independent predictors for unfavourable postoperative evolution in patients with aortic regurgitation undergoing aortic valve replacement. *Eur. Heart J.* **2009**, *30*, 865.
31. Matsumura, Y.; Hoshikawa-Nagai, E.; Kubo, T.; Yamasaki, N.; Furuno, T.; Kitaoka, H.; Takata, J.; Sugiura, T.; Doi, Y. Left ventricular reverse remodeling in long-term (>12 years) survivors with idiopathic dilated cardiomyopathy. *Am. J. Cardiol.* **2013**, *111*, 106–110. [CrossRef]
32. Iliuta, L. Predictors of persistent severe diastolic dysfunction after aortic valve replacement in aortic stenosis compared with aortic regurgitation. *Eur. Heart J.* **2012**, *33*, 667–668.
33. Iliuta, L.; Rac-Albu, M.; Rac-Albu, M.E.; Andronesi, A. Impact of Pulmonary Hypertension on Mortality after Surgery for Aortic Stenosis. *Medicina* **2022**, *58*, 1231. [CrossRef]
34. Diaconu, C. Cardiovascular complications of COVID-19. *Arch. Balk. Med. Union* **2021**, *56*, 139–141. [CrossRef]
35. Iliuta, L. Impact of Severe Pulmonary Hypertension on Outcomes Late After Aortic Valve Replacement for Aortic Stenosis Compared with Aortic Regurgitation. *Cardiology* **2014**, *128*, 177.
36. Ataç, A.; Kurt, E.; Yurdakul, S.E. An Overview to Ethical Problems in Telemedicine Technology. *Procedia Soc. Behav. Sci.* **2013**, *103*, 116–121. [CrossRef]

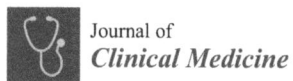

Article

Impact of SGLT2 Inhibitor Therapy on Right Ventricular Function in Patients with Heart Failure and Reduced Ejection Fraction

Ivona Mustapic [1,*,†], Darija Bakovic [1,2,†], Zora Susilovic Grabovac [1] and Josip A Borovac [1,3,4]

1. Cardiovascular Diseases Department, University Hospital of Split, 21000 Split, Croatia
2. Department of Physiology, University of Split School of Medicine, 21000 Split, Croatia
3. Department of Health Studies, University of Split, 21000 Split, Croatia
4. Department of Pathophysiology, University of Split School of Medicine, 21000 Split, Croatia
* Correspondence: mateljanka@gmail.com; Tel.: +385-95-2276-970
† These authors contributed equally to this work.

Abstract: Background: The impact of sodium-glucose cotransporter-2 inhibitors (SGLT2is) in addition to optimal medical therapy (OMT) on the right ventricular (RV) systolic function using advanced echocardiographic analysis among outpatients with heart failure and a reduced ejection fraction (HFrEF) has thus far been poorly investigated. **Methods:** This was a single-center, prospective, single-blinded study in which an echocardiographic expert was blinded to the allocation of the treatment. A total of 36 outpatients with HFrEF were randomized to either OMT or OMT+SGLT2i. Both groups underwent an echocardiographic examination of the RV systolic function at the baseline and at the 3-month follow-up (3mFU). **Results:** The patients in both groups did not significantly differ with respect to the relevant baseline comorbidities, therapy, and clinical characteristics. The patients receiving OMT+SGLT2i showed a significant improvement from the baseline to the 3mFU in all the measured RV echocardiographic parameters, while for the OMT group, a significant improvement after the 3mFU was observed for TAPSE and s'. The mean percent change from the baseline to the 3mFU was significant when comparing OMT+SGLT2i to the OMT group concerning RV FWS (+91% vs. +28%, $p = 0.039$), TR maxPG (−27% vs. +19%, $p = 0.005$), and TR Vmax (−17% vs. +13%, $p = 0.008$), respectively. **Conclusions:** Adding SGLT2i to OMT in patients with HFrEF resulted in a greater improvement in the RV systolic function from the baseline to the 3mFU compared to the OMT alone.

Keywords: SGLT2 inhibitors; right ventricular function; two-dimensional speckle tracking echocardiography; three-dimensional echocardiography; remodeling; heart failure with reduced ejection fraction

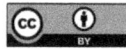

1. Introduction

Sodium-glucose co-transporter 2 inhibitors (SGLT2i) have emerged as a fundamental therapy for heart failure (HF) across the spectrum of ejection fractions. Recent results from the EMPEROR-Preserved and the DELIVER randomized trials have shown that SGLT2i (empagliflozin and dapagliflozin, respectively) can reduce all-cause mortality and hospitalizations due to HF in patients with HF with a mildly reduced or preserved ejection fraction [1,2]. The guidelines for the treatment of patients with heart failure with an reduced ejection fraction (HFrEF) by the European Society of Cardiology from September 2021 set SGLT2i as a pillar therapy with an IA class recommendation based on the results of the EMPEROR-Reduced and DAPA-HF trials [3–5].

The beneficial effects of SGLT2i on the left ventricular systolic and diastolic function, circulating natriuretic peptide levels, and functional symptom burden have been demonstrated in several studies, but not much is known about the effects of these drugs on the right ventricular (RV) systolic function [6,7]. The RV is often neglected because of its complex anatomy and the difficulty of obtaining satisfactory imaging "windows" in daily practice [8–10]. However, the RV has been shown to play an important prognostic role following cardiac surgery and in patients with HF, pulmonary arterial hypertension, or ischemic heart disease [11–13]. In clinical practice, the assessment of the RV function is usually undertaken by measuring only the longitudinal systolic function, as reflected in the measurement of the tricuspid annular plane systolic excursion (TAPSE) and tricuspid lateral annular systolic velocity (s' wave) derived from Doppler tissue imaging. The fractional area change (FAC), on the other hand, gives us an insight into the radial contraction of the RV [8]. Because these parameters are load- and angle-dependent, advanced echocardiographic methods, such as speckle-tracking echocardiography (STE) measuring the longitudinal strain of the RV free wall (RV FWS) and the three-dimensional RV ejection fraction (3D RVEF), have recently emerged as more accurate estimates of the RV systolic function [8,11]. The measurement of the 3D RVEF overcomes the limitations of the geometric assumption of the RV and integrates both the longitudinal and radial components of the myocardial muscle contraction, whereas TAPSE and s' wave measure only the longitudinal RV function in the basal region of the RV free wall [10]. The 3D echocardiography assessment of the RV ejection fraction and RV FWS have been shown to be comparable to the gold standard cardiac magnetic resonance (CMR) [11,14,15] and were shown to be an independent predictor of cardiac death and major adverse cardiovascular events (MACE) in patients with diverse cardiovascular diseases [14,16–18]. Furthermore, the ratio between the TAPSE and systolic pulmonary artery pressure (SPAP) represents the non-invasive measurement of the right ventriculo-arterial coupling and the RV contractile function [19].

For these reasons, we designed the present study to investigate the potential effects of SGLT2is on the RV systolic function after it was added to optimal medical therapy (OMT) for HFrEF.

2. Materials and Methods

2.1. Study Design, Inclusion, and Exclusion Criteria

This was a single-center, prospective, single-blinded study that was conducted from March 2021 to September 2021 at the Cardiovascular Disease Department, the University Hospital of Split, Croatia, in full compliance with the principles of the Declaration of Helsinki from 2013 and with the approval of the Ethics Committee of the University Hospital of Split under number 2181-147/01/06/M.S.-20-02. All the participants read and signed the informed consent form. We consecutively enrolled 36 outpatients with HFrEF according to the European Society of Cardiology guidelines (ESC) that were endorsed at the time of the initiation of the study (2016 edition) [20].

The inclusion criteria were: that the patients were diagnosed with HFrEF according to the ESC guidelines for the diagnosis and management of acute and chronic heart failure [20] and that they were aged 18 years or older with verified LVEF < 40%. At the time of inclusion, the patients were already required to receive background optimal guideline-directed medical therapy (OMT) at the highest tolerated daily doses of medications, including sacubitril-valsartan (angiotensin receptor neprilysin inhibitor—ARNi), beta-blocker (BB), and the mineralocorticoid receptor antagonist (MRA), in addition to other symptomatic therapies such as loop diuretics. In addition, only patients with a functional symptom severity class II and III, as assessed by the New York Heart Association (NYHA) scale, and a concurrent N-terminal-pro-b-type natriuretic peptide (NT-proBNP) value >125 pg/mL were included in the study.

Patients were excluded if they had: symptomatic hypotension (systolic blood pressure < 95 mmHg), an impaired renal function (eGFR < 30 mL/min/1.73 m^2 calculated according to the CKD-EPI formula) and serum potassium level > 5.2 mmol/L, hepatic dysfunction (defined as liver parameters such as ALT, AST, and/or ALP, which are three times above the upper 99-th percentile of the reference range, biliary cirrhosis and cholestasis, active malignancies (regardless of the stage and type of malignancy)), the current use of hormone replacement therapy, chemotherapy, or immunotherapy, the presence of an artificial heart valve (mechanical or biological), severe aortic stenosis, acute coronary syndrome in the three months preceding their enrollment in the study, percutaneous coronary intervention, or acute cerebrovascular incident in the last three months before the date of enrollment, pregnancy, or if they were breastfeeding. In addition, patients with diabetes mellitus treated with DPP4 inhibitors and GLP receptor agonists were excluded from the study because of possible interactions with the structure and function of the myocardial. Finally, patients who were unable to provide informed consent or declined to participate in the study were not enrolled.

After obtaining written informed consent, patients were consecutively randomized into two groups using a random number generator: (a) the OMT + SGLT2 inhibitor group (N = 18)—these patients received the SGLT2 inhibitor (either empagliflozin or dapagliflozin 10 mg once daily) in addition to background OMT—and (b) the OMT control group (N = 18); these patients received background OMT without the addition of SGLT2i. After their allocation to a therapy regimen, all patients were assigned to a standard and extended transthoracic echocardiographic (TTE) examination, physical examination, and biochemical laboratory testing at the baseline and the 3-month follow-up (3mFU).

Before the TTE examination, a detailed medical interview was performed regarding comorbidities, pharmacotherapy with daily doses for each treatment, their smoking status, and a physical examination with noninvasive measurements of taking their arterial blood pressure. The arterial blood pressure was determined as the mean of three consecutive measurements in the left antebrachial region. The functional NYHA status was determined in all patients. Peripheral venous blood samples for laboratory analyzes were collected on the morning of the examination day after overnight fasting and before the TTE examination. The samples were properly stored and analyzed by the same medical biochemistry specialist who was also blinded to the assignment of a treatment to the participants. All laboratory tests were performed according to good laboratory practice and included the measurement of the complete blood count (CBC), fasting plasma glucose, serum urea, creatinine, uric acid, electrolytes (sodium-Na, potassium-K), aspartate aminotransferase (AST), alanine, aminotransferase (ALT), gamma-glutamyl transferase (GGT), lactate dehydrogenase (LDH), C-reactive protein (CRP), and N-terminal-pro-brain natriuretic peptide (NT-proBNP) levels. The laboratory measurements were performed in all patients on the day of the first examination and repeated in the same fashion at the 3mFU.

2.2. Echocardiographic Examinations

All TTE examinations were performed with the patient at rest in the left supine position using the same commercially available ultrasound system (Vivid 9E, GE Medical System, Milwaukee, WI, USA). All the echocardiography data were digitally stored and analyzed on the Echo PAC workstation (Echo PAC 202 PC, GE Medical System, Milwaukee, USA).

The right ventricular systolic function was assessed with advanced TTE methods: two-dimensional STE evaluating the RV longitudinal strain of the RV free wall (RV FWS, −%) and three-dimensional RV ejection fraction (3D RVEF, %) using 3D echocardiography. The standard TTE parameters of the RV systolic function, such as the TAPSE, s' wave, and FAC, were also determined. The TAPSE measurement was performed in the apical 4-chamber view by directing the M-mode cursor to the lateral tricuspid annulus and was calculated as the total systolic displacement of the annular segment in millimeters [11]. From the same view, using the tissue Doppler (TD) cursor through the lateral tricuspid annulus in the basal segment of the RV free wall, the s' wave was calculated (cm/s), using the highest velocity of the systolic waveform [11]. In addition, from the apical 4-chamber view, the end-diastolic area (EDA) and end-systolic area (ESA) were calculated and the FAC was measured using the formula [(EDA − ESA)/EDA × 100] to obtain the percentage of the fractional area change. RV FWS was acquired from an RV focused apical 4-chamber view with an acquisition rate of 60 to 80 frames per second (fps) [11]. Using the two-dimensional STE of the three segments (the basal, middle, and apical segments) of the RV free wall, the mean peak systolic strain was measured by averaging the segmental peak values automatically generated by the software. The value of the RV FWS is expressed as a negative percentage because it represents longitudinal shortening, which is a reduction in the calculated speckle distance [18,21]. The example of "before–after" the RV FWS measurement is shown in Supplemental Figure S1.

To calculate the 3D RVEF, images were acquired with the 3D echo probe in apical four-chamber view using a pyramidal scan with a high image acquisition and wide-angle mode. The image was acquired in a cardiac cycle with 9 wedge-shaped subvolumes synchronized with electrocardiography while the patient held his breath for 7–10 s. The 3D RVEF measurement was performed at the workstation using EchoPAC software, with RV boundaries on the endomyocardium manually delineated and the RV volumes and ejection fraction automatically measured by the software [10,14]. The example of the 3D RVEF "before–after" measurement is shown in Supplemental Figure S2.

A color Doppler was placed over the tricuspid valve in the RV focused apical four-chamber view and a tricuspid regurgitation jet was defined. Then, using the continuous wave Doppler, the maximum tricuspid regurgitation velocity (TR Vmax, m/s) and the TR maximum pressure gradient (TR maXPG, mmHg) were calculated by tracing the TR spectrum. The systolic pulmonary artery pressure (SPAP) was calculated as the sum of the pressure gradient measured from the TR Vmax using the modified Bernoulli equation ($4\times$ (TR Vmax)2) and the right atrial pressure (mmHg) estimated on the basis of the inferior vena cava size and collapsibility during inspiration [22]. The ratio between the calculated values of the TAPSE and SPAP was then measured (mm/mmHg).

2.3. Outcome Measures

The primary endpoint was defined as the change in the RV systolic echocardiographic measurements (RV FWS, RV 3DEF, TAPSE, s' wave, FAC, TAPSE/SPAP, TR Vmax, and TR PPG) from the baseline to 3 months of continuous SGLT2i therapy combined with OMT in HFrEF patients.

The secondary endpoints were the differences in the mean percent change in the RV systolic echocardiographic measurement in patients receiving SGLT2i in addition to OMT compared with HfrEF patients receiving identical OMT without the addition of SGLT2i.

2.4. Sample Size Calculation

The sample size calculation and power analysis were conducted a priori by using the projected difference between the two independent means (the two groups of interest—OMT vs. OMT + SGLT2i). Left ventricular global longitudinal strain (LV GLS) is currently used in cardio-oncology as a tool to prevent cancer therapy-related cardiovascular toxicity and a significant change from the baseline to follow-up in patients receiving cancer-related therapy is defined as a 15% decrease in LV GLS from the baseline [23]. Because RV FWS has not been well studied, similar changes have not been described previously, but by analogy and considering the normal RV FWS value being greater than -19% [8], we defined a meaningful difference in the RV FWS between the two groups at the value of $2.0\% \pm 1.5\%$. These input parameters produced an effect size (d) of 1.33 with an alpha error (α) probability and statistical power (1-β error probability) defined at 0.05 and 0.95, respectively. Based on these assumptions, a total sample size of 26 patients was required for the study ($n = 13$ in each group).

2.5. Study Reliability

All the echocardiographic measurements were performed by the same cardiologist with a high level of expertise in echocardiography who was blinded to the allocation of a treatment to the participants. To reduce the intraobserver error, all the measurements from the beginning of the study were revised at the end of the study at the Echo PAC workstation. To reduce the interobserver error, the echocardiographic measurements were validated by another cardiology consultant with a high expertise in echocardiography to determine the possibility of a measurement error. The analysis of correlation and agreement between the expert echocardiographer assigned to the study and the control expert echocardiographer was performed by using Bland–Altman analysis and is available as Supplemental File S1.

2.6. Statistical Analysis

All the data analyses were performed by using SPSS Statistics for Windows, version 23.0 (IBM Corp., Armonk, NY, USA) and Prism, version 9.0.1. (Graphpad, La Jolla, CA, USA). Continuous data were, depending on the variable normality of distribution, shown as the mean ± standard deviation (SD) or median (interquartile range), while the categorical variables were displayed as whole numbers (N) and percentages (%). The normality of the data distribution was examined with the Kolmogorov–Smirnov test. The t-test for independent samples for variables with a normal distribution and Mann–Whitney U test for the variables with a non-normal distribution were utilized to measure the potential differences between the two groups of interest (OMT+SGLT2i vs. OMT group). The echocardiographic variables of interest were specifically examined in the "before–after" fashion in which the initial values (at the baseline) of each individual patient were pairwise compared to the values obtained at the follow-up. The mean absolute change (Δ, delta) in these values from the baseline to the 3mFU was reported for each group of interest and these values were compared between the groups by using a t-test. Similarly, for the purpose of a main analysis, the mean percent change from the baseline to the 3mFU was calculated for each group by using formula $[(Measurement_2 - Measurement_1)/Measurement_1] \times 100$ and these values were then compared between both groups by using an independent samples t-test. The Chi-squared (χ^2) test was used to examine the differences between the groups of interest with respect to the categorical variables, also for the measurements of the proportion of patients from each group that reached the cut-off value of RV FWS, which was 16% and above. Two-tailed significance values (p) were reported in all instances, while the results that reached $p < 0.05$ were considered to be statistically significant.

3. Results

3.1. Patients' Baseline Characteristics

A total of 36 consecutive HfrEF outpatients were randomized in the study. The baseline characteristics of the patients randomized to OMT+SLGT2i (n = 18) vs. OMT alone (n = 18) did not significantly differ concerning the age, sex, NYHA functional class, renal function, etiology of cardiomyopathy, relevant comorbidities (arterial hypertension, diabetes mellitus, dyslipidemia, and atrial fibrillation), and mean daily dose or distribution of the chronic HF-related therapies, as it can be appreciated from Table 1. Importantly, all the patients in both groups received the identical background OMT consisting of ARNi, BB, and MRA.

Table 1. Baseline characteristics of two treatment groups (OMT vs. OMT + SGLT2 inhibitor).

Variable	OMT (n = 18)	OMT + SGLT2i (n = 18)	p-Value *
Age, years	67.8 ± 12.7	67.3 ± 11.5	0.902
Male sex, %	16 (88.9)	16 (88.9)	1.000
NYHA functional class	2.2 ± 0.38	2.3 ± 0.49	0.371
Smoking, %	6 (33.3)	8 (44.4)	0.494
Dyslipidemia, %	11 (61.1)	10 (55.6)	0.735
Arterial hypertension, %	13 (72.2)	14 (77.8)	0.700
Diabetes mellitus, %	4 (22.2)	7 (38.9)	0.154
Atrial fibrillation, %	7 (38.8)	5 (27.8)	0.297
Ischemic cardiomyopathy, %	9 (50.0)	6 (33.3)	0.310
Systolic blood pressure, mmHg	123 ± 18	124 ± 19	0.860
Diastolic blood pressure, mmHg	73 ± 10	74 ± 14	0.782
Heart rate, bpm	81 ± 21	80 ± 25	0.965
3D LVEF, %	28.5 ± 8.5	30.2 ± 9.7	0.573
LV GLS, %	−7.8 ± 3.8	−7.8 ± 3.7	0.965
LVEDV, mL	223 ± 71	236 ± 85	0.609
LVESV, mL	139 ± 67	145 ± 72	0.782

Table 1. Cont.

Variable	OMT (n = 18)	OMT + SGLT2i (n = 18)	p-Value *
LA volume, mL	81 ± 36	81 ± 27	0.988
E/E'	13.6 ± 5.2	13.8 ± 5.5	0.901
MV E/A	1.21 ± 0.7	1.12 ± 0.5	0.647
AV V$_{max}$, m/s	1.18 ± 0.35	1.17 ± 0.31	0.968
PVAT, msec	122 ± 32	120 ± 30	0.907
Hemoglobin, g/L	146 ± 15	144 ± 14	0.632
Fasting glucose, mmol/L	6.2 ± 2.1	6.8 ± 1.6	0.377
eGFR, mL/min./1.73 m^2	64 ± 19	70 ± 17	0.295
Sodium, mmol/L	139 ± 2.0	138 ± 3.1	0.802
Potassium, mmol/L	4.4 ± 0.5	4.5 ± 0.8	0.772
C-reactive protein, mg/L	4.2 (0.9–7.2)	2.4 (1.0–6.9)	0.743
NT-proBNP, pg/mL	2326 (1188–5191)	3250 (1463–6227)	0.606
AST, IU/L	28 (25–36)	27 (23–33)	0.323
ALT, IU/L	39 ± 26	35 ± 14	0.544
GGT, IU/L	49 ± 32	67 ± 49	0.202
LDH, IU/L	191 (180–243)	206 (180–236)	0.864
ARNi + BB + MRA at baseline, %	18 (100)	18 (100)	1.000
Furosemide use, %	10 (55.6)	10 (55.6)	1.000
Statin use, %	10 (55.6)	10 (55.6)	1.000
Oral anticoagulant use, %	9 (50.0)	9 (50.0)	1.000
Sacubril-valsartan daily dose, mg	250 ± 115	239 ± 110	0.768
Beta-blocker daily dose, mg	3.75 ± 1.9	3.61 ± 1.3	0.803
MRA daily dose, mg	34.7 ± 12.5	33.3 ± 12.1	0.738
Furosemide daily dose, mg	61.4 ± 78.8	57.0 ± 91.3	0.886

Abbreviations: AV V$_{max}$—aortic valve peak velocity; ALT—alanine aminotransferase; ARNi—angiotensin receptor neprilysin inhibitor; AST—aspartate aminotransferase; BB—beta blocker; E/A—peak velocity blood flow in early diastole to peak velocity blood flow in late diastole ratio; E/E'—early mitral inflow velocity to mitral annular early diastolic velocity ratio; eGFR—estimated glomerular filtration rate calculated by CKD-EPI formula; GGT—gama-glutamyl transferase; GLS-global longitudinal strain; LA—left atrium; LDH—lactate dehydrogenase; LVEDV-left ventricular end-diastolic volume; LVESV—left ventricular end-systolic volume; LVEF—left ventricular ejection fraction; MRA—mineralocorticoid receptor antagonist; NT-proBNP—N-terminal pro brain natriuretic peptide; PVAT—pulmonary velocity acceleration time; NYHA—New York Heart Association; * Results are presented as n (percent) and analyzed through Chi-squared test, mean ± standard deviation (t-test of independent samples) or median (interquartile range) analyzed through Mann–Whitney U test, based on variable normality.

Furthermore, both groups did not significantly differ with respect to the baseline laboratory indices while they were similar in the baseline echocardiographic parameters reflecting the left ventricular systolic and diastolic function (Table 1).

In both of the examined groups, the echocardiographic parameters of the right ventricular systolic function were predominantly reduced, however, the obtained values measured at the baseline echocardiographic examination were similar in both groups (Table 2).

3.2. Absolute Mean Changes in Advanced Echocardiographic Parameters of Right Ventricular Function in Each Treatment Group, from Baseline to 3mFU

Patients with HfrEF randomized to the OMT+SGLT2i treatment experienced a significant improvement from the baseline to the 3mFU in all the RV functional echocardiographic parameters that were measured, as reflected in the mean absolute change, as follows: TAPSE (+4.5 mm, $p = 0.002$), s' (+3.5 cm/s, $p = 0.032$), 3D RVEF (+10.1%, $p = 0.003$), RV FWS (+7.2%, $p < 0.001$), and RV FAC (+9.0%, $p = 0.029$). On the other hand, the improvement from the baseline to the 3mFU in the OMT-only group was significant only for the TAPSE and s' wave (+2.4 mm, $p = 0.040$ and +2.7 cm/s, $p = 0.013$, respectively), while the 3D RVEF, RV FWS, and RV FAC were all associated with a numerical improvement but failed to reach a statistical significance (Table 3).

Table 2. Right-sided functional echocardiographic parameters at baseline, stratified by the type of treatment received (OMT vs. OMT + SGLT2 inhibitor).

Variable	OMT (n = 18)	OMT + SGLT2i (n = 18)	p-Value *
TAPSE, mm	10.4 ± 3.7	9.2 ± 3.4	0.404
s′, cm/s	9.7 ± 4.5	11.1 ± 5.5	0.447
3D RVEF, %	38.8 ± 10.2	38.6 ± 8.5	0.936
RV FWS, %	−15.2 ± 5.6	−17.2 ± 6.3	0.488
FAC, %	34 ± 13	37 ± 14	0.462
TR maxPG, mmHg	22.7 ± 16.7	29.0 ± 19.2	0.290
TR V_{max}, m/s	2.2 ± 0.9	2.6 ± 1.0	0.287
TAPSE/SPAP, mm/mHg	0.76 ± 0.70	0.76 ± 1.02	0.977

Abbreviations: FAC—fractional area change; RV—right ventricle; RV FWS—right ventricular free wall strain; TAPSE—tricuspid annular plane systolic excursion; TAPSE/SPAP—tricuspid annular plane systolic excursion/systolic pulmonary artery pressure; s′-tissue Doppler velocity of the basal free lateral wall of the right ventricle; TR maxPG—tricuspid regurgitant maximum pressure gradient; TR V_{max}—tricuspid regurgitation max jet velocity; 3D RVEF—3D right ventricular ejection fraction. * Results are presented as mean ± standard deviation (t-test of independent samples).

Table 3. Absolute changes in values of right-sided functional echocardiographic parameters at baseline and 3-month follow-up, stratified by the type of treatment received (OMT vs. OMT + SGLT2 inhibitor).

Variable	OMT (n = 18)				OMT + SGLT2i (n = 18)			
	Baseline	3-Month Follow-Up	Δ Change Absolute	p-Value	Baseline	3-Month Follow-Up	Δ Change Absolute	p-Value
TAPSE, mm	10.4 ± 3.7	12.8 ± 5.0	+2.4	0.040 *	9.2 ± 3.4	13.7 ± 3.5	+4.5	0.002 *
s′, cm/s	9.7 ± 4.5	12.4 ± 5.4	+2.7	0.013 *	11.1 ± 5.5	14.6 ± 5.0	+3.5	0.032 *
3D RVEF, %	38.8 ± 10.2	42.3 ± 10.3	+3.5	0.432	38.6 ± 8.5	48.7 ± 9.8	+10.1	0.003 *
RV FWS, %	−15.2 ± 5.6	−18.5 ± 6.7	+3.3	0.067	−17.2 ± 6.3	−24.4 ± 5.8	+7.2	<0.001 *
RV FAC, %	34 ± 13	35.0 ± 10.8	+1.8	0.686	37 ± 14	46 ± 9	+9.0	0.029 *
TR maxPG, mmHg	22.7 ± 16.7	24.2 ± 16.0	+1.5	0.679	29.0 ± 19.2	17.6 ± 12.3	−11.5	0.002 *
TR V_{max}, m/s	2.2 ± 0.9	2.5 ± 1.4	+0.3	0.248	2.6 ± 1.0	1.9 ± 0.7	−0.7	0.003 *
TAPSE/SPAP, mm/mmHg	0.76 ± 0.70	0.92 ± 1.04	+0.16	0.605	0.76 ± 1.02	1.39 ± 1.07	+0.63	0.079

Abbreviations: RV FAC—right ventricular fractional area change; RV—right ventricle; RV FWS—right ventricular free wall strain; TAPSE—tricuspid annular plane systolic excursion; TAPSE/SPAP—tricuspid annular plane systolic excursion/systolic pulmonary artery pressure; s′—tissue Doppler velocity of the basal free lateral wall of the right ventricle; TR maxPG—tricuspid regurgitant maximum pressure gradient; TR V_{max}—tricuspid regurgitation max jet velocity; 3D RVEF—3D right ventricular ejection fraction. * Two-tailed significance values (p) were reported in all instances, while the results that reached $p < 0.05$ were considered to be statistically significant.

The echocardiographic parameters measuring the tricuspid regurgitation maximal velocity (TR V_{max}) and maximum pressure gradient (TR maxPG) were significantly reduced from the baseline to the 3mFU in patients that were randomized to the OMT+SGLT2i treatment (−0.7 m/s, $p = 0.003$ and −11.5 mmHg, $p = 0.002$, respectively). Contrary to this, no significant changes regarding the tricuspid regurgitation echocardiographic parameters were observed in the patients randomized only to OMT (Table 3). The TAPSE/SPAP ratio did not differ between the groups at the baseline (Table 2), and both groups showed no improvement after the 3mFU with a greater improvement in the OMT+SGLT2i group compared with the OMT-control group but without a statistical significance (Table 3).

3.3. Mean Percent Change in Echocardiographic Parameters of RV Systolic Function between OMT+SGLT2i and OMT Groups, from Baseline to 3mFU

The analysis directly comparing the mean percent change (%) from the baseline to the 3mFU demonstrated a greater numerical improvement for all the RV systolic function parameters in the OMT+SGLT2i vs. OMT group, however, a statistical significance was reached only for RV FWS, TR V_{max}, and TR maxPG (Figure 1). It is of note that the addition of SGLT2i to OMT was associated with a mean 63% increase in the RV FWS compared to the OMT-only group (Figure 1A), while a tricuspid regurgitation was significantly more reduced in the OMT+SGLT2i group compared to the OMT-only group (46% reduction in TR maxPG and 30% reduction in TR V_{max}, Figure 1B,C, respectively).

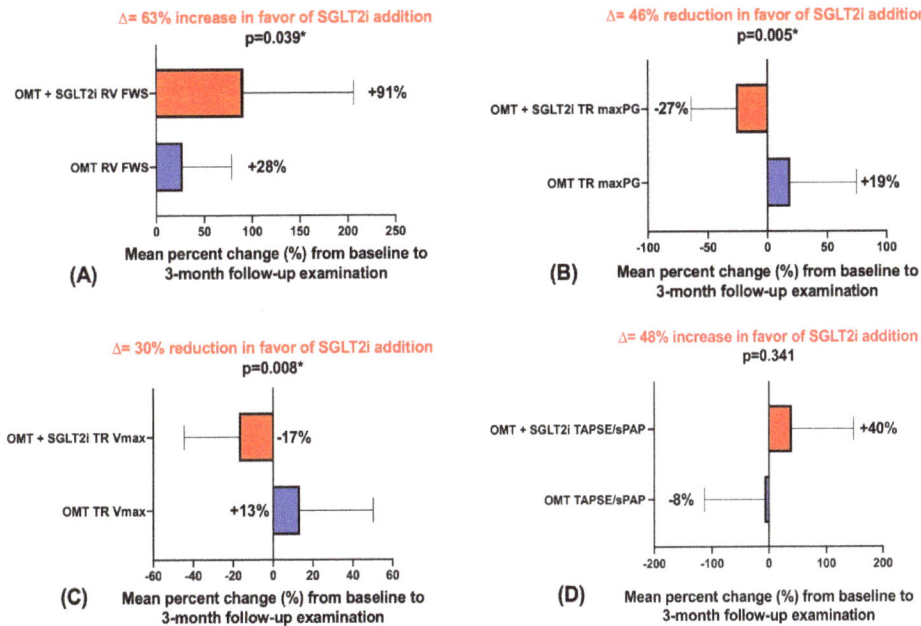

Figure 1. Mean percent change (%) from baseline to 3-month follow-up; red—OMT+SGLT2i group, blue—OMT control group; (**A**)—mean percent change in right ventricular free wall strain between groups from baseline to 3mFU; (**B**)—mean percent change in TR maximal pressure gradient between groups from baseline to 3mFU; (**C**)—mean percent change in maximal TR velocity between groups from baseline to 3mFU; (**D**)—mean percent change in TAPSE/SPAP ratio between groups from baseline to 3mFU. * Two-tailed significance values (p) were reported in all instances, while the results that reached $p < 0.05$ were considered to be statistically significant.

The TAPSE/SPAP ratio showed a mean percent increase of 48% from the baseline to the 3mFU in favor of the OMT+SGLT2i+ group compared with the OMT-group, but did not reach a statistical significance when comparing between the groups (Figure 1D).

Furthermore, TAPSE showed 47% ($p = 0.084$) a greater improvement from the baseline to the 3mFU in favor of the OMT+SGLT2i treatment, the s' wave increased by 8% ($p = 0.769$) in the OMT+SGLT2i group, the FAC increased by the mean of 25% ($p = 0.477$) in the OMT+SGLT2i group, and the 3D RVEF increased by 15% more in the OMT+SGLT2i ($p = 0.345$) compared to the OMT-only group (Figure 2A–D, respectively).

When combined together and averaged, the global improvement in the RV hemodynamics encompassing all the measured RV systolic parameters yielded an average $33 \pm 10\%$ improvement in the OMT+SGLT2i group compared to the OMT-only group, from the baseline to the 3 mFU ($p = 0.006$, Supplemental Figure S3).

Finally, as demonstrated in Figure 3, a group of patients that had SGLT2i added to OMT had a significantly lesser proportion of impaired RV FWS ($\leq 16\%$) at the 3 mFU, compared to patients that received OMT only (11.1% vs. 44.4%, $p = 0.026$).

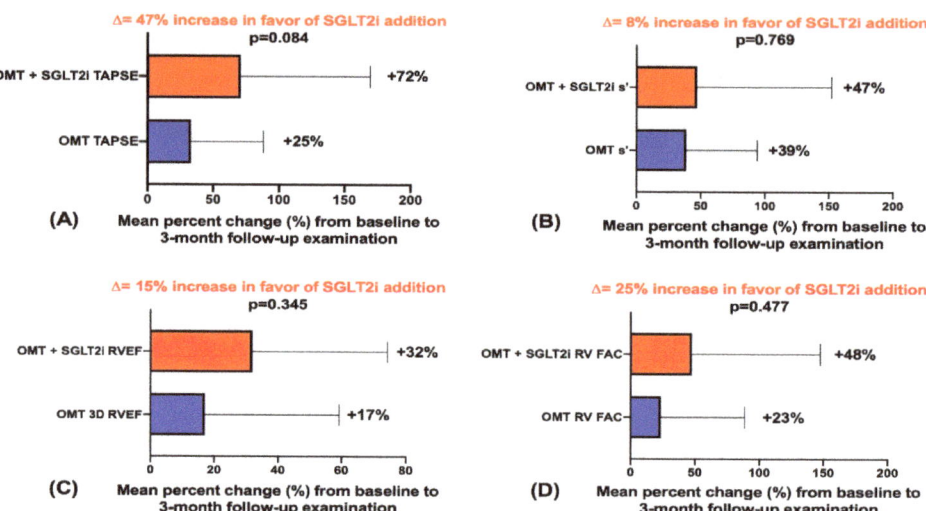

Figure 2. Mean percent change (%) from baseline to 3-month follow-up; red—OMT+SGLT2i group, blue—OMT control group; (**A**)—mean percent change in tricuspid annular plane systolic excursion (TAPSE) between groups from baseline to 3mFU; (**B**)—mean percent change in Doppler tissue imaging-derived tricuspid lateral annular systolic velocity (s' wave) between groups from baseline to 3mFU; (**C**)—mean percent change in right ventricular ejection fraction measured by three-dimensional echocardiography between groups from baseline to 3mFU; (**D**)—mean percent change in fractional area change (FAC) between groups from baseline to 3mFU.

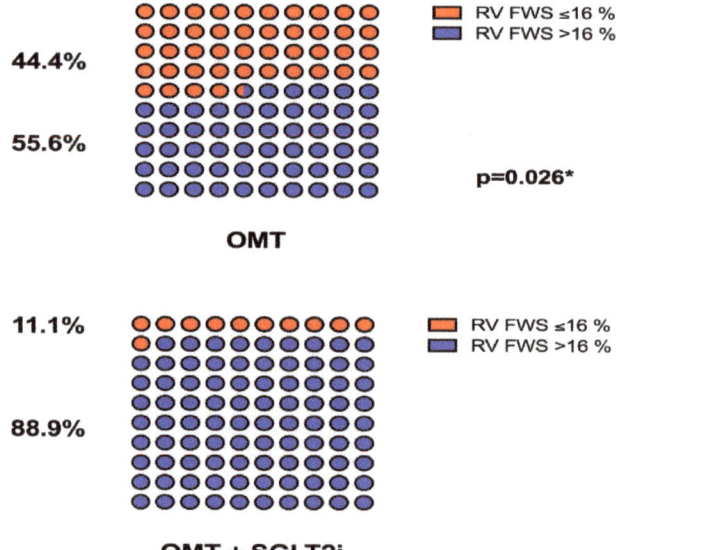

Figure 3. Upper image—proportion of patients from the OMT control group with the right ventricular free wall strain value (RV FWS) of −16% or more positive to absolute zero value (red color); or above −16% and more negative value from absolute zero value. Bottom image—proportion of patients from the OMT+ SGLT2i+ group with the right ventricular free wall strain value (RV FWS) of −16% or more positive to absolute zero (red color); or over −16% and more negative value from absolute zero.

It should also be noted that the echocardiographic measurements at the baseline and the 3mFU visit showed a low degree of discrepancy between the expert sonographer responsible for all the measurements undertaken in the study and the control expert sonographer (results in Supplemental File S1).

4. Discussion

In this prospective study in which consecutive outpatients with HFrEF were randomly allocated to a treatment group, we demonstrated an echocardiographic improvement in the RV systolic function from the baseline to the follow-up visit at 3 months among the patients that had SGLT2i added to OMT compared to those that received OMT only. Furthermore, the addition of SGLT2i to OMT appeared to significantly reduce the degree of tricuspid regurgitation compared to a treatment with OMT alone.

The exact effects of SGLT2i on the RV function have not been thus far studied in great detail. Patoulias and colleagues emphasized the need to evaluate the effects of SGLT2i on the RV function, citing the RV as a "forgotten" cardiac chamber with significant knowledge gaps [7]. A post hoc analysis of the EMPA-HEART CardioLink-6 trial in patients with type II diabetes mellitus and coronary artery disease (CAD) showed no differences in the RV mass index, RV volume, and RV EF, measured by CMR after 6 months of empagliflozin compared with placebo [24]. Conversely to this, a recent retrospective study demonstrated a significant improvement in the pulmonary artery's stiffness and RV systolic function in HFrEF patients after 6 months of SGLT2i therapy compared to the baseline, as measured by TAPSE, s' wave, and FAC, along with a significant decrease in the mean pulmonary systolic pressure [25]. However, to the best of our knowledge, our study is the first one that prospectively examined the effects of an SGLT2i addition to OMT in HFrEF outpatients on the RV systolic function using advanced 3D echocardiography and 2D speckle-tracking of the RV free wall.

It is important to emphasize that our results were obtained in groups that were well matched on many relevant baseline covariates. All of the patients in both groups received the same OMT, which was maximally up-titrated to the individual patient and consisted of foundational HFrEF therapy with ARNi, BB, MRA, and furosemide. There were no differences between the groups in the average daily dose of the therapies. No therapy was titrated or suspended during the follow-up period because the participating patients had already received the maximum tolerated therapy. More importantly, the included HFrEF population did not differ in either the systolic or diastolic left ventricular function and had similar values of LV GLS and LV 3DEF.

Mouton and colleagues emphasized a cut-off value of RV FWS < −16% for the diagnosis of the RV systolic dysfunction with a high specificity and moderate sensitivity for poor outcomes in the HFrEF population [26]. Our results showed that 4 times fewer patients in the OMT+SGLT2i group had RV FWS ≤ −16% than patients only receiving OMT alone. Moreover, RV FWS is not only a prognostic parameter but is also able to detect the subtle deterioration of the RV systolic function despite the preserved TAPSE, s' wave, and FAC in HF patients [27,28]. Another important feature of RV FWS is that it likely reflects the extent of RV myocardial fibrosis in the later stages of HFrEF development [29]. These observations are important in the context of our results, as our study showed a numerical improvement in all the measured parameters of the RV systolic function from the baseline to the 3mFU in patients receiving SGLT2i in addition to OMT, however, RV FWS was the only echocardiographic indicator that was statistically significant improved compared to the OMT-only group.

Thus far, studies on the impact of ARNi in HFrEF patients showed an improvement in left and right ventricular function [30,31]. According to a recent meta-analysis, ARNi improves the right ventricular function and reduces the pulmonary hypertension independent of the left ventricular reverse remodeling [32–34]. In our study, all the enrolled patients were taking ARNi as the background therapy in maximally uptitrated doses that were tolerated by the patients. The group of patients not receiving SGLT2i after 3 months of a follow-up showed a numerical improvement in all the measured RV parameters, but only the TAPSE and s' wave reached a statistical significance, which is in accordance with previous studies [31].

The results of the EMBRACE-HF study focused on HF patients in a wide spectrum of LVEF and regardless of the DM status with NYHA class III-IV and the pulmonary arterial hypertension (mean diastolic pulmonary artery pressure(PAP) of 22 mmHg) showed that PAP was reduced with empagliflozin compared with the placebo after 12 weeks of therapy, but the effects on the RV were not studied [35]. Previously, studies using animal models have shown a reduction in the mean PAP under SGLT2i therapy and a reduction in the RV hypertrophy [24,36,37]. The results of our study clearly show the same signal, as there was a highly statistically significant reduction in the TR Vmax and TR maxPG from the baseline to the 3mFU in patients receiving SGLT2i in addition to maximally uptitrated OMT, whereas these parameters remained similar after the 3mFU in patients receiving maximally uptitrated OMT alone. Importantly, a significantly greater reduction in the tricuspid regurgitation parameters was retained when OMT+SGLT2i and OMT-only groups were directly compared. It should be emphasized that patients in both groups had a similar degree of RV systolic dysfunction, mild tricuspid regurgitation, and a low probability of pulmonary hypertension calculated by TAPSE/SPAP at the baseline [38]. The estimate of TAPSE/SPAP has a high predictive value and correlates with the stiffness of the pulmonary artery [39,40], which is important given our results of a greater improvement from the baseline to the 3mFU in patients receiving SGLT2i comparing to OMT-only patients.

The exact pathophysiological mechanisms explaining these results waits to be elucidated. However, the beneficial role of SGLT2i in reducing the extent of pulmonary hypertension and RV remodeling can be explained by their multifactorial and pleiotropic effects. SGLT2i have metabolic, vascular, and hemodynamic effects. They reduce body weight due to a renal caloric loss by glycosuria, have beneficial effects on the cardiac metabolism, and improve the cardiac energetics [41]. They also reduce myocardial oxidative stress, and by inhibiting the myocardial sodium-hydrogen exchanger 1 (NHE1), they the reduce cytoplasmic sodium and calcium levels [41,42]. The combination of the different mechanisms prevents cardiac remodeling. Due to the mechanism of osmotic diuresis, the initial volume depletion results in a decrease in the pulmonary pressure within the first few days after the initiation of the treatment [35]. The patients in our study did not differ in terms of the average diuretic dose, so the possible explanation for the SGLT2i effect is the addition of the osmotic diuretic and natriuretic effects, which led to a reduction in the RV preload. In addition, SGLT2 inhibitors attenuate the activation of the renin-angiotensin-aldosterone system (RAAS) and reduce the discharge of the sympathetic nervous system, which in turn attenuates systemic and pulmonary arterial stiffening [34,35,43]. Camci and Yilmaz demonstrated the beneficial role of SGLT2i in reducing the pulmonary arterial stiffness (PAS) wherefore patients exhibit a better pulmonary vascular compliance, which attenuates the RV afterload and thus improves the RV systolic function [25]. Additionally, the previously demonstrated reduction in the LV filling pressure and improvement in the LV diastolic function is reflected in the improvement in the RV function [6,44]. Another beneficial effect of SGLT2i that may explain the improvement in the RV is its action on vascular cells through an anti-inflammatory and antioxidant effect, also increasing the angiogenesis and nitric oxide bioavailability from the endothelium, leading to pulmonary and systemic vasodilation, thereby reducing the RV preload and afterload [45,46].

There are some limitations to our work that should be noted. This was a single-center study enrolling an ethnically homogeneous population, thus these observations might not be able to be generalized to the overall or worldwide population. Furthermore, given that this was a "concept-generating" study that enrolled a rather small number of HFrEF patients, it is possible that some of the presented results would reach a statistical significance if a larger number of patients was enrolled. It is also possible that a timeframe greater than 3 months and a longer follow-up might be required to show a greater benefit of the addition of SGLT2i to background OMT for the improvement in the RV function in HFrEF. Similarly, a low number of patients might have generated random differences that could impact on the obtained results. Our study was not powered nor designed to capture clinical outcomes such as death and/or hospitalization events, although we can state that all patients were well-compensated at their second examination and none of them died or required hospitalization within 1 year from the follow-up examination based on our follow-up records. However, the strengths of this study are that both of the compared groups were well-matched in important baseline covariates and were treated with the same background OMT that was, correspondingly, nearly identical with respect to the daily doses. Finally, the patients were consecutively enrolled and randomly allocated a treatment, while all the measurements were recorded by the single sonographer with a high expertise in advanced echocardiography who was blinded to the allocation of the treatment. Last but not least, the echocardiographic measurements were validated against another expert sonographer.

5. Conclusions

This concept-generating study demonstrated that among outpatients with HFrEF, the addition of SGLT2i to maximally uptitrated OMT resulted in a significant improvement in the RV systolic function from the baseline to the 3mFU. Moreover, a significant improvement among the OMT+SGLT2i vs. OMT-only patients was demonstrated in the parameters of the RV free wall strain and the parameters reflecting the degree of tricuspid regurgitation. Taken together, our results suggest that the addition of SGLT2i to background OMT provides an incremental benefit concerning the RV hemodynamics in outpatients with HFrEF. Further large-scale studies are welcome and warranted to confirm these initial findings.

Supplementary Materials: The following supporting information can be downloaded at: https://www.mdpi.com/article/10.3390/jcm12010042/s1, File S1: The analysis of correlation and agreement between the expert echocardiographer assigned to the study and the control expert echocardiographer performed by using Bland–Altman analysis. Figure S1: The advanced echocardiographic measurement of right ventricular free wall strain at the (a) baseline and (b) 3-month follow-up examination; Figure S2: The advanced echocardiographic measurement of right ventricular 3D ejection fraction and other structural/functional parameters at the (a) baseline and (b) 3-month follow-up examination; Figure S3: Mean percent change (%) improvement in RV hemodynamics, encompassing all measured RV systolic parameters, from the baseline to 3mFU between the two groups.; red—OMT+SGLT2i group, blue—OMT control group.

Author Contributions: Conceptualization, I.M. and D.B.; methodology, I.M. and J.A.B.; validation, I.M., D.B., and J.A.B.; formal analysis, J.A.B.; investigation, I.M., D.B. and Z.S.G.; resources, J.A.B.; data curation, I.M. and J.A.B.; writing—original draft preparation, I.M. and D.B.; writing—review and editing, I.M., D.B., Z.S.G. and J.A.B.; visualization, J.A.B.; supervision, I.M. and J.A.B. All authors have read and agreed to the published version of the manuscript.

Funding: This research received no external funding.

Institutional Review Board Statement: The study was conducted from March 2021 to September 2021 at the Clinic for Heart and Vascular Diseases, University Hospital of Split, Croatia. All procedures performed in studies with human participants were in accordance with the principles of the 2013 Declaration of Helsinki and were approved by the Ethics Committee of the University Hospital of Split filed under the number 2181-147/01/06/M.S.-20-02.

Informed Consent Statement: Informed consent was obtained from all subjects involved in the study.

Data Availability Statement: Data sets generated and/or analyzed during the current study are available on reasonable request from the corresponding author.

Conflicts of Interest: The authors declare no conflict of interest.

References

1. Anker, S.D.; Butler, J.; Filippatos, G.; Ferreira, J.P.; Bocchi, E.; Bohm, M.; Brunner-La Rocca, H.P.; Choi, D.J.; Chopra, V.; Chuquiure-Valenzuela, E.; et al. Empagliflozin in Heart Failure with a Preserved Ejection Fraction. *N. Engl. J. Med.* **2021**, *385*, 1451–1461. [CrossRef] [PubMed]
2. Solomon, S.D.; McMurray, J.J.V.; Claggett, B.; de Boer, R.A.; DeMets, D.; Hernandez, A.F.; Inzucchi, S.E.; Kosiborod, M.N.; Lam, C.S.P.; Martinez, F.; et al. Dapagliflozin in Heart Failure with Mildly Reduced or Preserved Ejection Fraction. *N. Engl. J. Med.* **2022**, *387*, 1089–1098. [CrossRef] [PubMed]
3. Packer, M.; Anker, S.D.; Butler, J.; Filippatos, G.; Pocock, S.J.; Carson, P.; Januzzi, J.; Verma, S.; Tsutsui, H.; Brueckmann, M.; et al. Cardiovascular and Renal Outcomes with Empagliflozin in Heart Failure. *N. Engl. J. Med.* **2020**, *383*, 1413–1424. [CrossRef] [PubMed]
4. McMurray, J.J.V.; Solomon, S.D.; Inzucchi, S.E.; Kober, L.; Kosiborod, M.N.; Martinez, F.A.; Ponikowski, P.; Sabatine, M.S.; Anand, I.S.; Belohlavek, J.; et al. Dapagliflozin in Patients with Heart Failure and Reduced Ejection Fraction. *N. Engl. J. Med.* **2019**, *381*, 1995–2008. [CrossRef]
5. McDonagh, T.A.; Metra, M.; Adamo, M.; Gardner, R.S.; Baumbach, A.; Böhm, M.; Burri, H.; Butler, J.; Čelutkienė, J.; Chioncel, O.; et al. 2021 ESC Guidelines for the diagnosis and treatment of acute and chronic heart failure. *Eur. Heart J.* **2021**, *42*, 3599–3726. [CrossRef] [PubMed]
6. Lan, N.S.R.; Fegan, P.G.; Yeap, B.B.; Dwivedi, G. The effects of sodium-glucose cotransporter 2 inhibitors on left ventricular function: Current evidence and future directions. *ESC Heart Fail.* **2019**, *6*, 927–935. [CrossRef]
7. Patoulias, D.; Katsimardou, A.; Toumpourleka, M.; Papadopoulos, C.; Doumas, M. Time to assess the effects of sodium-glucose co-transporter-2 inhibitors on the 'forgotten' right ventricle? *ESC Heart Fail.* **2020**, *7*, 337–338. [CrossRef]
8. Lee, J.H.; Park, J.H. Strain Analysis of the Right Ventricle Using Two-dimensional Echocardiography. *J. Cardiovasc. Imaging* **2018**, *26*, 111–124. [CrossRef]
9. Kovács, A.; Lakatos, B.; Tokodi, M.; Merkely, B. Right ventricular mechanical pattern in health and disease: Beyond longitudinal shortening. *Heart Fail. Rev.* **2019**, *24*, 511–520. [CrossRef]
10. Ahmad, A.; Li, H.; Zhang, Y.; Liu, J.; Gao, Y.; Qian, M.; Lin, Y.; Yi, L.; Zhang, L.; Li, Y.; et al. Three-Dimensional Echocardiography Assessment of Right Ventricular Volumes and Function: Technological Perspective and Clinical Application. *Diagnostics* **2022**, *12*, 806. [CrossRef]
11. Smolarek, D.; Gruchala, M.; Sobiczewski, W. Echocardiographic evaluation of right ventricular systolic function: The traditional and innovative approach. *Cardiol. J.* **2017**, *24*, 563–572. [CrossRef] [PubMed]
12. Ayach, B.; Fine, N.M.; Rudski, L.G. Right ventricular strain: Measurement and clinical application. *Curr. Opin. Cardiol.* **2018**, *33*, 486–492. [CrossRef]
13. Tadic, M.; Nita, N.; Schneider, L.; Kersten, J.; Buckert, D.; Gonska, B.; Scharnbeck, D.; Reichart, C.; Belyavskiy, E.; Cuspidi, C.; et al. The Predictive Value of Right Ventricular Longitudinal Strain in Pulmonary Hypertension, Heart Failure, and Valvular Diseases. *Front. Cardiovasc. Med.* **2021**, *8*, 698158. [CrossRef] [PubMed]
14. Nagata, Y.; Wu, V.C.; Kado, Y.; Otani, K.; Lin, F.C.; Otsuji, Y.; Negishi, K.; Takeuchi, M. Prognostic Value of Right Ventricular Ejection Fraction Assessed by Transthoracic 3D Echocardiography. *Circ. Cardiovasc. Imaging* **2017**, *10*, e005384. [CrossRef] [PubMed]
15. Ishizu, T.; Seo, Y.; Atsumi, A.; Tanaka, Y.O.; Yamamoto, M.; Machino-Ohtsuka, T.; Horigome, H.; Aonuma, K.; Kawakami, Y. Global and Regional Right Ventricular Function Assessed by Novel Three-Dimensional Speckle-Tracking Echocardiography. *J. Am. Soc. Echocardiogr.* **2017**, *30*, 1203–1213. [CrossRef]
16. Iacoviello, M.; Citarelli, G.; Antoncecchi, V.; Romito, R.; Monitillo, F.; Leone, M.; Puzzovivo, A.; Lattarulo, M.S.; Rizzo, C.; Caldarola, P.; et al. Right Ventricular Longitudinal Strain Measures Independently Predict Chronic Heart Failure Mortality. *Echocardiography* **2016**, *33*, 992–1000. [CrossRef]
17. Houard, L.; Benaets, M.B.; de Meester de Ravenstein, C.; Rousseau, M.F.; Ahn, S.A.; Amzulescu, M.S.; Roy, C.; Slimani, A.; Vancraeynest, D.; Pasquet, A.; et al. Additional Prognostic Value of 2D Right Ventricular Speckle-Tracking Strain for Prediction of Survival in Heart Failure and Reduced Ejection Fraction: A Comparative Study With Cardiac Magnetic Resonance. *JACC Cardiovasc. Imaging* **2019**, *12*, 2373–2385. [CrossRef] [PubMed]
18. Ji, M.; Wu, W.; He, L.; Gao, L.; Zhang, Y.; Lin, Y.; Qian, M.; Wang, J.; Zhang, L.; Xie, M.; et al. Right Ventricular Longitudinal Strain in Patients with Heart Failure. *Diagnostics* **2022**, *12*, 445. [CrossRef]
19. Kazimierczyk, R.; Kazimierczyk, E.; Knapp, M.; Sobkowicz, B.; Malek, L.A.; Blaszczak, P.; Ptaszynska-Kopczynska, K.; Grzywna, R.; Kaminski, K.A. Echocardiographic Assessment of Right Ventricular-Arterial Coupling in Predicting Prognosis of Pulmonary Arterial Hypertension Patients. *J. Clin. Med.* **2021**, *10*, 2995. [CrossRef]
20. Ponikowski, P.; Voors, A.A.; Anker, S.D.; Bueno, H.; Cleland, J.G.F.; Coats, A.J.S.; Falk, V.; González-Juanatey, J.R.; Harjola, V.P.; Jankowska, E.A.; et al. 2016 ESC Guidelines for the diagnosis and treatment of acute and chronic heart failure: The Task Force for the diagnosis and treatment of acute and chronic heart failure of the European Society of Cardiology (ESC)Developed with the special contribution of the Heart Failure Association (HFA) of the ESC. *Eur. Heart J.* **2016**, *37*, 2129–2200. [CrossRef]

21. Badano, L.P.; Kolias, T.J.; Muraru, D.; Abraham, T.P.; Aurigemma, G.; Edvardsen, T.; D'Hooge, J.; Donal, E.; Fraser, A.G.; Marwick, T.; et al. Standardization of left atrial, right ventricular, and right atrial deformation imaging using two-dimensional speckle tracking echocardiography: A consensus document of the EACVI/ASE/Industry Task Force to standardize deformation imaging. *Eur. Heart J. Cardiovasc. Imaging* **2018**, *19*, 591–600. [CrossRef] [PubMed]
22. Parasuraman, S.; Walker, S.; Loudon, B.L.; Gollop, N.D.; Wilson, A.M.; Lowery, C.; Frenneaux, M.P. Assessment of pulmonary artery pressure by echocardiography—A comprehensive review. *Int. J. Cardiol. Heart Vasc.* **2016**, *12*, 45–51. [CrossRef] [PubMed]
23. Lyon, A.R.; Lopez-Fernandez, T.; Couch, L.S.; Asteggiano, R.; Aznar, M.C.; Bergler-Klein, J.; Boriani, G.; Cardinale, D.; Cordoba, R.; Cosyns, B.; et al. 2022 ESC Guidelines on cardio-oncology developed in collaboration with the European Hematology Association (EHA), the European Society for Therapeutic Radiology and Oncology (ESTRO) and the International Cardio-Oncology Society (IC-OS). *Eur. Heart J.* **2022**, *43*, 4229–4361. [CrossRef]
24. Sarak, B.; Verma, S.; David Mazer, C.; Teoh, H.; Quan, A.; Gilbert, R.E.; Goodman, S.G.; Bami, K.; Coelho-Filho, O.R.; Ahooja, V.; et al. Impact of empagliflozin on right ventricular parameters and function among patients with type 2 diabetes. *Cardiovasc. Diabetol.* **2021**, *20*, 200. [CrossRef]
25. Camci, S.; Yilmaz, E. Effects of Sodium-Glucose Co-Transporter-2 Inhibition on Pulmonary Arterial Stiffness and Right Ventricular Function in Heart Failure with Reduced Ejection Fraction. *Medicina* **2022**, *58*, 1128. [CrossRef] [PubMed]
26. Mouton, S.; Ridon, H.; Fertin, M.; Pentiah, A.D.; Goémine, C.; Petyt, G.; Lamblin, N.; Coisne, A.; Foucher-Hossein, C.; Montaigne, D.; et al. 2D-speckle tracking right ventricular strain to assess right ventricular systolic function in systolic heart failure. Analysis of the right ventricular free and posterolateral walls. *Int. J. Cardiol.* **2017**, *245*, 190–195. [CrossRef]
27. Morris, D.A.; Krisper, M.; Nakatani, S.; Kohncke, C.; Otsuji, Y.; Belyavskiy, E.; Radha Krishnan, A.K.; Kropf, M.; Osmanoglou, E.; Boldt, L.H.; et al. Normal range and usefulness of right ventricular systolic strain to detect subtle right ventricular systolic abnormalities in patients with heart failure: A multicentre study. *Eur. Heart J. Cardiovasc. Imaging* **2017**, *18*, 212–223. [CrossRef]
28. Carluccio, E.; Biagioli, P.; Alunni, G.; Murrone, A.; Zuchi, C.; Coiro, S.; Riccini, C.; Mengoni, A.; D'Antonio, A.; Ambrosio, G. Prognostic Value of Right Ventricular Dysfunction in Heart Failure With Reduced Ejection Fraction: Superiority of Longitudinal Strain Over Tricuspid Annular Plane Systolic Excursion. *Circ. Cardiovasc. Imaging* **2018**, *11*, e006894. [CrossRef]
29. Lisi, M.; Cameli, M.; Righini, F.M.; Malandrino, A.; Tacchini, D.; Focardi, M.; Tsioulpas, C.; Bernazzali, S.; Tanganelli, P.; Maccherini, M.; et al. RV Longitudinal Deformation Correlates With Myocardial Fibrosis in Patients With End-Stage Heart Failure. *JACC Cardiovasc. Imaging* **2015**, *8*, 514–522. [CrossRef]
30. Zandstra, T.E.; Nederend, M.; Jongbloed, M.R.M.; Kies, P.; Vliegen, H.W.; Bouma, B.J.; Tops, L.F.; Schalij, M.J.; Egorova, A.D. Sacubitril/valsartan in the treatment of systemic right ventricular failure. *Heart* **2021**, *107*, 1725–1730. [CrossRef]
31. Bouali, Y.; Galli, E.; Paven, E.; Laurin, C.; Arnaud, H.; Oger, E.; Donal, E. Impact of sacubitril/valsartan on systolic heart failure: Right heart location and clustering analysis. *Adv. Clin. Exp. Med.* **2022**, *31*, 109–119. [CrossRef] [PubMed]
32. Zhang, J.; Du, L.; Qin, X.; Guo, X. Effect of Sacubitril/Valsartan on the Right Ventricular Function and Pulmonary Hypertension in Patients With Heart Failure With Reduced Ejection Fraction: A Systematic Review and Meta-Analysis of Observational Studies. *J. Am. Heart Assoc.* **2022**, *11*, e024449. [CrossRef] [PubMed]
33. Yang, Y.; Shen, C.; Lu, J.; Fu, G.; Xiong, C. Sacubitril/Valsartan in the Treatment of Right Ventricular Dysfunction in Patients With Heart Failure With Reduced Ejection Fraction: A Real-world Study. *J. Cardiovasc. Pharmacol.* **2022**, *79*, 177–182. [CrossRef] [PubMed]
34. King, N.E.; Brittain, E. Emerging therapies: The potential roles SGLT2 inhibitors, GLP1 agonists, and ARNI therapy for ARNI pulmonary hypertension. *Pulm. Circ.* **2022**, *12*, e12028. [CrossRef]
35. Nassif, M.E.; Qintar, M.; Windsor, S.L.; Jermyn, R.; Shavelle, D.M.; Tang, F.; Lamba, S.; Bhatt, K.; Brush, J.; Civitello, A.; et al. Empagliflozin Effects on Pulmonary Artery Pressure in Patients With Heart Failure: Results From the EMBRACE-HF Trial. *Circulation* **2021**, *143*, 1673–1686. [CrossRef]
36. Chowdhury, B.; Luu, A.Z.; Luu, V.Z.; Kabir, M.G.; Pan, Y.; Teoh, H.; Quan, A.; Sabongui, S.; Al-Omran, M.; Bhatt, D.L.; et al. The SGLT2 inhibitor empagliflozin reduces mortality and prevents progression in experimental pulmonary hypertension. *Biochem. Biophys. Res. Commun.* **2020**, *524*, 50–56. [CrossRef]
37. Tang, Y.; Tan, S.; Li, M.; Tang, Y.; Xu, X.; Zhang, Q.; Fu, Q.; Tang, M.; He, J.; Zhang, Y.; et al. Dapagliflozin, sildenafil and their combination in monocrotaline-induced pulmonary arterial hypertension. *BMC Pulm. Med.* **2022**, *22*, 142. [CrossRef]
38. Humbert, M.; Kovacs, G.; Hoeper, M.M.; Badagliacca, R.; Berger, R.M.F.; Brida, M.; Carlsen, J.; Coats, A.J.S.; Escribano-Subias, P.; Ferrari, P.; et al. 2022 ESC/ERS Guidelines for the diagnosis and treatment of pulmonary hypertension. *Eur. Heart J.* **2022**, *43*, 3618–3731. [CrossRef]
39. Grignola, J.C.; Domingo, E.; Lopez-Meseguer, M.; Trujillo, P.; Bravo, C.; Perez-Hoyos, S.; Roman, A. Pulmonary Arterial Remodeling Is Related to the Risk Stratification and Right Ventricular-Pulmonary Arterial Coupling in Patients With Pulmonary Arterial Hypertension. *Front. Physiol.* **2021**, *12*, 631326. [CrossRef]
40. Vicenzi, M.; Caravita, S.; Rota, I.; Casella, R.; Deboeck, G.; Beretta, L.; Lombi, A.; Vachiery, J.L. The added value of right ventricular function normalized for afterload to improve risk stratification of patients with pulmonary arterial hypertension. *PLoS ONE* **2022**, *17*, e0265059. [CrossRef]
41. Seferović, P.M.; Fragasso, G.; Petrie, M.; Mullens, W.; Ferrari, R.; Thum, T.; Bauersachs, J.; Anker, S.D.; Ray, R.; Çavuşoğlu, Y.; et al. Sodium-glucose co-transporter 2 inhibitors in heart failure: Beyond glycaemic control. A position paper of the Heart Failure Association of the European Society of Cardiology. *Eur. J. Heart Fail.* **2020**, *22*, 1495–1503. [CrossRef] [PubMed]

42. Verma, S.; McMurray, J.J.V. SGLT2 inhibitors and mechanisms of cardiovascular benefit: A state-of-the-art review. *Diabetologia* **2018**, *61*, 2108–2117. [CrossRef] [PubMed]
43. Madonna, R. Exploring the mechanisms of action of gliflozines in heart failure and possible implications in pulmonary hypertension. *Vascul. Pharmacol.* **2021**, *138*, 106839. [CrossRef]
44. Pabel, S.; Hamdani, N.; Singh, J.; Sossalla, S. Potential Mechanisms of SGLT2 Inhibitors for the Treatment of Heart Failure With Preserved Ejection Fraction. *Front. Physiol.* **2021**, *12*, 752370. [CrossRef] [PubMed]
45. Durante, W.; Behnammanesh, G.; Peyton, K.J. Effects of Sodium-Glucose Co-Transporter 2 Inhibitors on Vascular Cell Function and Arterial Remodeling. *Int. J. Mol. Sci.* **2021**, *22*, 8786. [CrossRef]
46. Juni, R.P.; Kuster, D.W.D.; Goebel, M.; Helmes, M.; Musters, R.J.P.; van der Velden, J.; Koolwijk, P.; Paulus, W.J.; van Hinsbergh, V.W.M. Cardiac Microvascular Endothelial Enhancement of Cardiomyocyte Function Is Impaired by Inflammation and Restored by Empagliflozin. *JACC Basic Transl. Sci.* **2019**, *4*, 575–591. [CrossRef]

Disclaimer/Publisher's Note: The statements, opinions and data contained in all publications are solely those of the individual author(s) and contributor(s) and not of MDPI and/or the editor(s). MDPI and/or the editor(s) disclaim responsibility for any injury to people or property resulting from any ideas, methods, instructions or products referred to in the content.

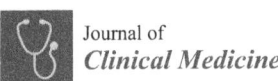

Article

Association between Remote Dielectric Sensing and Estimated Plasma Volume to Assess Body Fluid Distribution

Teruhiko Imamura [1,*,†], Toshihide Izumida [1,†], Nikhil Narang [2], Hiroshi Onoda [1], Masaki Nakagaito [1], Shuhei Tanaka [1], Makiko Nakamura [1], Ryuichi Ushijima [1], Hayato Fujioka [1], Kota Kakeshita [1] and Koichiro Kinugawa [1]

[1] Second Department of Internal Medicine, University of Toyama, Toyama 930-0194, Japan
[2] Advocate Christ Medical Center, Oak Lawn, IL 60453, USA
* Correspondence: teimamu@med.u-toyama.ac.jp; Tel.: +81-76-434-2281; Fax: +81-76-434-5026
† These authors contributed equally to the work.

Abstract: Background: Pulmonary congestion is quantified by a remote dielectric sensing (ReDS^{TM}) system, while systemic congestion is estimated by calculated plasma volume. The type of clinical patient profile as defined by the ReDS system and calculated plasma volume remains uncertain. Methods: Hospitalized patients with or without heart failure were included in this prospective study. On admission, ReDS values were measured and plasma volume status (PVS) was estimated using their body weight at the same time. Cutoffs of ReDS value and PVS were defined at 34% and −2.7%, respectively. The association between the two parameters was assessed. Results: A total of 482 patients (median 76 years, 288 men) were included. The median ReDS value was 28% (25%, 32%) and median PVS was −16.4% (−26.3%, −5.9%). Of the patients, 64 had high ReDS value (and low PVS) and 80 had high PVS (and low ReDS value). The high ReDS group had a higher prevalence of clinical heart failure with a more elevated echocardiographic E/e′ ratio, whereas the high PVS group had a higher prevalence of chronic kidney disease ($p < 0.05$ for all). Four out of a total of six patients with high ReDS value and high PVS had both heart failure and chronic kidney disease profiles. Conclusion: The combination of ReDS value and PVS was able to clinically stratify the types of body fluid distribution and patient profiles. Utilizing these tools may assist the clinician in constructing a therapeutic strategy for the at-risk hospitalized patient.

Keywords: congestion; heart failure; hemodynamics

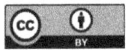

1. Introduction

In patients with chronic heart failure, residual pulmonary and systemic congestion following attempts at medical optimization is associated with an increased risk of morbidity and mortality [1]. Nevertheless, the practical and non-invasive tools that can accurately quantify the degree of pulmonary and systemic congestion in daily clinical practice are limited. Clinical examination often cannot accurately estimate pulmonary and systemic congestion compared to invasive right heart catheterization. It should be noted that routinely performing invasive hemodynamic assessments is not feasible for the majority of institutions that care for patients with heart failure [2].

The remote dielectric sensing (ReDS^{TM}, Sensible Medical Innovations Ltd., Netanya, Israel) system is a non-invasive electro-magnetic technology that quantifies the degree of pulmonary congestion within one minute of application and without needing a high level of technical expertise [3]. ReDS values, whose normal range is suggested between 20% and 35%, have been shown to have a moderate correlation (i.e., approximate r value of 0.6) with other modalities, including chest-computed tomography and pulmonary capillary wedge pressure [4–6].

Recently, a novel technique to non-invasively estimate plasma volume (PV) using hematocrit (Ht) and body weight (BW), has been made commercially available [7]. PV is considered to represent the amount of extra-vascular fluid. This modality was validated using scintigraphy tests and the ability to accurately estimate systemic congestion has been shown in recently published clinical studies [8,9].

The association between ReDS and PV quantification has not been rigorously analyzed thus far. The combination of these two methods may prove effective in assessing total body volume distribution, allowing the clinician to construct therapeutic strategies for each patient. In this study, we evaluated the volume distribution profile of hospitalized patients with cardiovascular diseases using both the ReDS system and estimated PV.

2. Methods

2.1. Participant Selection

Patients who were hospitalized for treatment of their cardiovascular diseases including heart failure were considered to be included in this cross-sectional study. Patients were assumed to have heart failure when they had a history of heart failure or ongoing heart failure, which was diagnosed by Framingham's criteria, irrespective of their left ventricular ejection fraction. Chronic kidney disease was defined as estimated glomerular filtration ratio <60 mL/min/1.73 m^2 or urinary albumin excretion ≥300 mg/day.

On admission, ReDS measurements were performed as detailed below. PV was calculated as detailed below using Ht and BW data on admission.

Patients who were unable to wear an ReDS system due to body size (for example, body mass index > 35), or those with lung pathology including pneumonia and lung cancer, were not eligible to undergo ReDS measurements. Patients who had BW data that was not collected on admission were also excluded. Informed consent was obtained from all participants beforehand. The institutional ethical review board approved the study protocol.

2.2. ReDS Measurement

ReDS measurements were performed on all participants. ReDS employs low-power electromagnetic signals emitted between two sensors embedded on a wearable device and can quantify lung fluid amount within one minute non-invasively with normal breathing mechanics [3]. The manufacturer-proposed normal range for the ReDS value is between 25% and 34%.

2.3. PV Estimation

All participants received BW, body height, and Ht measurements on admission. The PV was estimated by calculating the Hakim formula: PV (L) = [1 − Ht (%)] × [a × (b × (lean body mass))], in which a = 1530 for males and 864 for females, and b = 41.0 for males and 47.2 for females. The lean body mass was calculated as follows: 0.33 × BW (kg) + 0.34 × [body height (cm)] − 29.5 for males and 0.30 × BW (kg) + 0.42 × [body height (cm)] − 43.3 for females [7].

PV status (PVS) was calculated as follows: PVS (%) = [((estimated PV) − (ideal PV))/(ideal PV)] × 100. Ideal PV (L) = a × BW (kg), in which a = 39 for males and 40 for females.

2.4. Other Variables

Laboratory data including plasma B-type natriuretic peptide and transthoracic echocardiography data were obtained on admission according to the standard manner.

2.5. Statistical Methods

Continuous variables were calculated as a median and interquartile range. Categorical variables were calculated as numbers and percentages. The correlation between ReDS values and estimated PVS was assessed using Pearson's correlation.

A cutoff of ReDS value was defined at 34%. Patients with ReDS values above this cutoff were classified as having clinically significant pulmonary congestion. A cutoff of PVS was defined at −2.7% [10]. Although a definite cutoff of PVS has not yet been established, the mean value of PVS in the healthy cohort was −2.7%. Patients with a PVS above this cutoff were assumed to have significant systemic congestion. Patients were stratified into four groups using these two cutoffs for both ReDS and PVS.

All analyses were performed in SPSS Statistics 23.0 software (IBM Corp, Armonk, NY, USA), and two-tailed p values less than 0.05 were assumed to be significant.

3. Results

3.1. Baseline Characteristics

A total of 500 hospitalized patients were considered for study inclusion. Of these, 18 patients with pneumonia were excluded. Eventually, 482 patients were included in the final study cohort. Median age was 76 (69, 82) years old and 288 (60%) were men (Table 1). Of these, 136 (28%) had a diagnosis of heart failure (including 33 preserved ejection fraction) and 319 (66%) had chronic kidney disease.

Table 1. Baseline characteristics.

	Total (N = 482)	High ReDS and/or High PVS (N = 150)	Low ReDS and Low PVS (N = 332)	p Value
Demographics				
Age, years	76 (69, 82)	77 (71, 84)	76 (68, 81)	0.021 *
Men	288 (60%)	106 (71%)	182 (55%)	0.001 *
Body mass index	22.8 (20.5, 25.2)	21.3 (18.8, 23.8)	23.3 (21.4, 25.8)	<0.001 *
Systolic blood pressure, mmHg	123 (106, 137)	120 (102, 136)	125 (108, 138)	0.15
Heart rate, bpm	73 (65, 84)	74 (66, 83)	72 (65, 84)	0.89
Comorbidity				
Heart failure	136 (28%)	50 (33%)	86 (26%)	0.059
Hypertension	356 (74%)	115 (77%)	241 (73%)	0.20
Dyslipidemia	264 (55%)	80 (53%)	184 (55%)	0.37
Diabetes mellitus	170 (35%)	66 (44%)	104 (31%)	0.005 *
Chronic obstructive pulmonary disease	21 (4%)	7 (5%)	14 (4%)	0.32
Persistent atrial fibrillation	77 (16%)	21 (14%)	55 (17%)	0.47
Paroxysmal atrial fibrillation	94 (20%)	31 (21%)	61 (18%)	0.55
Chronic kidney disease	319 (66%)	106 (71%)	213 (64%)	0.097
History of stroke	90 (19%)	32 (21%)	58 (17%)	0.19
History of coronary intervention	115 (24%)	43 (29%)	72 (22%)	0.062
Valvular disease	160 (33%)	68 (45%)	92 (28%)	<0.001 *
Laboratory data				
Hemoglobin, g/dL	12.6 (11.2, 13.9)	11.9 (10.2, 13.0)	13.0 (11.5, 14.2)	<0.001 *
Serum albumin, g/dL	3.9 (3.6, 4.2)	3.7 (3.4, 4.0)	3.9 (3.7, 4.2)	<0.001 *
Serum GOT, IU/L	24 (12, 33)	27 (13, 35)	23 (12, 34)	0.076
Serum GPT, IU/L	23 (11, 34)	25 (12, 34)	22 (11, 33)	0.068
Serum creatinine, mg/mL	1.0 (0.8, 1.5)	1.1 (0.8, 2.0)	1.0 (0.9, 1.3)	0.002 *
Serum sodium, mg/dL	140 (138, 141)	139 (137, 141)	140 (138, 141)	0.28
Plasma B-type natriuretic peptide, pg/mL	105 (35, 283)	174 (71, 498)	84 (27, 196)	<0.001 *
Echocardiography				
Left ventricular end-diastolic diameter, mm	48 (44, 55)	49 (44, 57)	48 (44, 54)	0.15
Left ventricular ejection fraction, %	63 (51, 71)	62 (50, 71)	63 (52, 72)	0.70
Left atrial diameter, mm	41 (35, 50)	43 (35, 52)	41 (35, 49)	0.072
E/e' ratio	8.5 (6.2, 9.8)	11.2 (9.5, 12.9)	7.6 (5.6, 9.2)	0.013 *
ReDS value, %	28 (25, 32)	32 (25, 38)	28 (25, 31)	<0.001 *
Plasma volume status, %	−16.4 (−26.3, −5.9)	−1.5 (−19.5, 6.1)	−18.7 (−27.6, −11.7)	<0.001 *

Continuous variables are stated as median (25% interquartile, 75% interquartile) and compared between the two groups using the Mann–Whitney U test. Categorical variables are stated as numbers and percentage and compared between the two groups using Fischer's exact test. * $p < 0.05$. GOT, glutamate oxaloacetate transaminase; GPT, glutamate pyruvate transaminase; ReDS, remote dielectric sensing; PVS, plasma volume status.

3.2. Association between ReDS Value and PVS

Median ReDS value was 28% (25%, 32%) and median PVS was −16.4% (−26.3%, −5.9%). These values were distributed widely (Figure 1A,B). There was a significant but weak correlation between the two values ($r = -0.20$, $p < 0.001$; N = 482; Figure 2). Of these, 70 patients had ReDS values >34% and 86 patients had PVS >−2.7%. Most of the patients

(69%) had a low ReDS value and low PVS. Only six patients had a high ReDS value and high PVS.

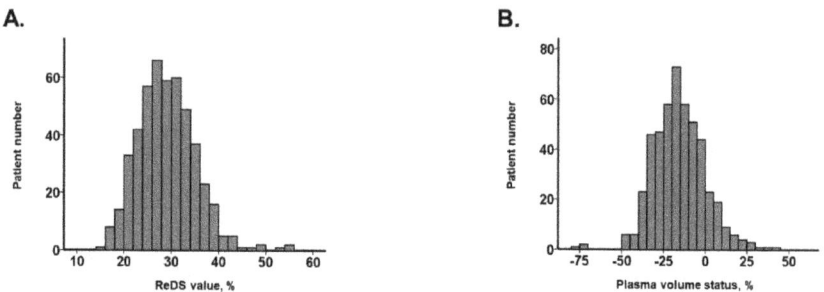

Figure 1. Distribution of ReDS value (A) and PVS (B).

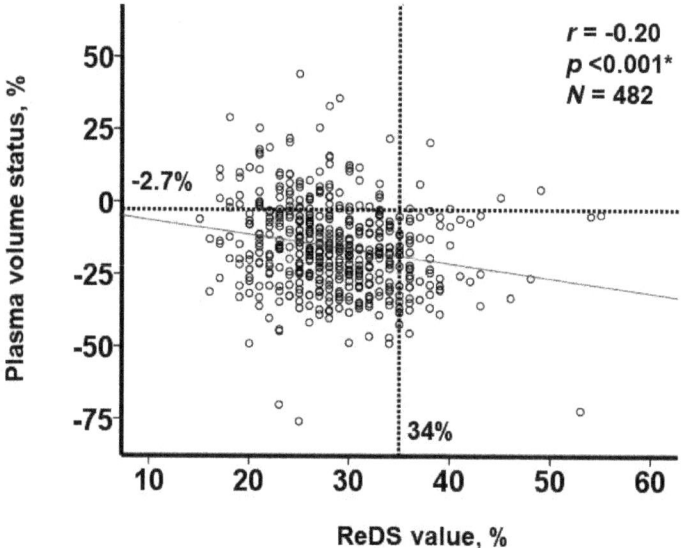

Figure 2. Correlation between ReDS value and PVS. Cutoffs for ReDS value and PVS were defined at 34% and −2.7%, respectively. * $p < 0.05$ by Pearson's correlation.

3.3. Profile of Those with High ReDS Value and/or High PVS

Out of all the patients, 150 (31%) had a high ReDS value and/or high PVS. They tended to have heart failure (33% versus 26%) and chronic kidney disease (71% versus 64%) more frequently than those with a low ReDS value and low PVS ($p = 0.059$ and $p = 0.097$, respectively; Table 1). They also had a higher plasma level of B-type natriuretic peptide and a higher echocardiographic E/e' ratio than those with a low ReDS value and low PVS ($p < 0.001$ and $p = 0.013$, respectively). They also had higher prevalence of diabetes mellitus, anemia, and hypoalbuminemia than those with a low ReDS value and low PVS ($p < 0.05$ for all).

3.4. Profile Comparison between High ReDS Group and High PVS Group

Out of all the patients, 64 had a high ReDS value (and low PVS) and 80 had a high PVS (and low ReDS value) (Figure 2). The high ReDS group was younger and had a more elevated echocardiographic E/e' ratio than the high PVS group ($p < 0.05$ for both; Table 2). The high PVS group was older and had a higher prevalence of chronic kidney disease than the high ReDS group ($p < 0.05$ for all; Table 2). They also had a higher prevalence of anemia, hypoalbuminemia, and a higher plasma B-type natriuretic peptide level than the high ReDS group ($p < 0.05$ for all).

Table 2. Comparison between high ReDS group and high PVS group.

	High ReDS (N = 64)	High PVS (N = 80)	p Value
Demographics			
Age, years	73 (63, 82)	79 (73, 84)	0.002 *
Men	35 (55%)	66 (83%)	<0.001 *
Body mass index	24.3 (21.9, 28.6)	19.4 (17.6, 20.8)	<0.001 *
Systolic blood pressure, mmHg	121 (104, 137)	119 (102, 139)	0.78
Heart rate, bpm	77 (64, 90)	70 (65, 82)	0.16
Comorbidity			
Heart failure	21 (33%)	25 (31%)	0.49
Hypertension	44 (69%)	66 (83%)	0.042 *
Dyslipidemia	33 (52%)	44 (55%)	0.40
Diabetes mellitus	24 (38%)	38 (48%)	0.15
Chronic obstructive pulmonary disease	3 (5%)	4 (5%)	0.67
Persistent atrial fibrillation	11 (17%)	10 (13%)	0.67
Paroxysmal atrial fibrillation	17 (27%)	14 (18%)	0.37
Chronic kidney disease	38 (59%)	63 (79%)	0.010 *
History of stroke	12 (19%)	18 (23%)	0.37
History of coronary intervention	16 (25%)	25 (31%)	0.26
Valvular disease	26 (41%)	39 (49%)	0.21
Laboratory data			
Hemoglobin, g/dL	12.6 (11.2, 13.6)	11.2 (10.1, 12.4)	<0.001 *
Serum albumin, g/dL	3.9 (3.5, 4.2)	3.7 (3.3, 3.9)	0.012 *
Serum GOT, IU/L	26 (14, 34)	29 (14, 41)	0.076
Serum GPT, IU/L	24 (13, 33)	27 (13, 38)	0.066
Serum creatinine, mg/mL	0.9 (0.7, 1.4)	1.5 (0.9, 3.9)	<0.001 *
Serum sodium, mg/dL	140 (138, 142)	139 (137, 141)	0.18
Plasma B-type natriuretic peptide, pg/mL	124 (63, 422)	216 (93, 501)	0.034 *
Echocardiography			
Left ventricular end-diastolic diameter, mm	49 (45, 58)	48 (43, 57)	0.59
Left ventricular ejection fraction, %	62 (52, 71)	65 (50, 72)	0.59
Left atrial diameter, mm	44 (37, 54)	41 (34, 51)	0.24
E/e' ratio	12.1 (10.2, 13.6)	9.8 (7.7, 10.6)	0.025 *
ReDS value, %	37 (36, 39)	25 (21, 28)	<0.001 *
Plasma volume status, %	−24.0 (−31.3, −12.2)	5.1 (0.6, 11.4)	<0.001 *

Continuous variables are stated as median (25% interquartile, 75% interquartile) and compared between the two groups using the Mann–Whitney U test. Categorical variables are stated as numbers and percentage and compared between the two groups using Fischer's exact test. * $p < 0.05$. GOT, glutamate oxaloacetate transaminase; GPT, glutamate pyruvate transaminase; ReDS, remote dielectric sensing; PVS, plasma volume status.

3.5. Profile of Patients with High ReDS and High PVS

Only six patients had a high ReDS and high PVS (median 78 [73, 87] years old, five men). Of these, four patients (67%) had both heart failure and chronic kidney disease and one patient had chronic kidney disease alone. Median ReDS value was 39% (37%, 45%) and median PVS was 2.9% (−2.2%, 6.1%). Median echocardiographic E/e' ratio was 13.2 (10.7, 14.7) and median serum creatinine was 3.0 (0.9, 5.0) mg/dL.

3.6. Profile of Patients with and without Heart Failure

Several key parameters were compared between those with and without heart failure (Table 3). Plasma B-type natriuretic peptide levels and echocardiographic E/e' ratio were higher in the heart failure group, whereas ReDS values and PVS were not statistically different between the two groups.

Table 3. Comparison between those with and without heart failure.

	Heart Failure (N = 136)	No Heart Failure (N = 346)	p Value
Serum creatinine, mg/mL	1.1 (0.8, 1.5)	1.0 (0.8, 1.4)	<0.001 *
Plasma B-type natriuretic peptide, pg/mL	293 (116, 591)	80 (26, 208)	<0.001 *
E/e' ratio	10.4 (8.4, 12.2)	9.1 (7.7, 10.9)	0.008 *
ReDS value, %	28 (25, 34)	29 (25, 33)	0.30
Plasma volume status, %	−17.1 (−25.6, −4.4)	−15.8 (−25.7, −7.4)	0.18

Continuous variables are stated as median (25% interquartile, 75% interquartile) and compared between the two groups using Mann–Whitney U test. * $p < 0.05$. ReDS, remote dielectric sensing; PVS, plasma volume status.

Among 136 heart failure patients, ReDS values did not have any correlations with ejection fraction ($p = 0.15$) and B-type natriuretic peptide levels ($p = 0.11$). The PVS did not have correlation with ejection fraction ($p = 0.30$), but had a significant but weak correlation with B-type natriuretic peptide ($p = 0.032$, r = 0.18).

4. Discussion

We investigated patients' profiles stratified by ReDS values and PVS among those who were hospitalized for treatment for cardiovascular diseases. The high ReDS (and low PVS) group had a more elevated echocardiographic E/e' ratio, whereas the high PVS (and low ReDS) group had a higher prevalence of chronic kidney disease. Four out of six patients satisfying both a high ReDS value and high PVS had both heart failure and chronic kidney disease.

4.1. Rationale for Utilizing ReDS System and PVS

Assessment of pulmonary congestion can be challenging. The ReDS system can quantify the degree of pulmonary congestion with reasonable accuracy when compared to other modalities, including high-resolution computed tomography [5], right heart catheterization [4], and lung ultrasound [11].

The methodology to estimate the PVS by using the Hakim formula, as a surrogate of systemic congestion, was demonstrated and validated by previous studies [8,9]. Its prognostic impact was demonstrated in cohorts of patients with severe aortic stenosis [12], ischemic heart disease requiring coronary artery bypass surgery [13], and advanced heart failure requiring a durable left ventricular assist device [14]. Given the clinical conditions where quantifying systemic congestion was observed to be feasible, we sought to estimate a comprehensive congestion profile in a cohort with a low likelihood of clinical congestion in addition to those who have a higher likelihood of a clinically abnormal congestion profile.

4.2. Patients' Profiles Stratified by ReDS Value and PVS

No positive correlation existed between ReDS values and PVS. ReDS values overall did not have a strong correlation with PVS. Thus, ReDS cannot be an alternative to PVS, and vice versa. In other words, the combination of both modalities may be more practical to accurately understand body fluid distribution than each alone.

Patients' clinical profiles were uniquely characterized by combination of both modalities. Patients with a high ReDS value had a higher prevalence of heart failure etiology and a more elevated echocardiographic E/e' ratio. The elevations of intra-cardiac filling pressures due to impaired cardiac function often coincide with pulmonary congestion, though may not manifest as systemic congestion [15]. Prior analyses have shown that ReDS value moderately correlates with pulmonary capillary artery pressure, but does not strongly correlate with central venous pressure [4].

Patients with a high PVS tended to have chronic kidney disease and a lower echocardiographic E/e' ratio. These patients may therefore have systemic volume overload due to impaired renal function [16], and may not have pulmonary congestion. They had higher plasma B-type natriuretic peptide levels than those with high ReDS, probably due to a higher prevalence of chronic kidney disease in this cohort.

4.3. Clinical Implication

A combination of both modalities may be practical to estimate patients' profiles and determine therapeutic strategy, instead of either modality alone, particularly at the time of admission when comprehensive clinical assessments ha not yet been completed.

When ReDS values are high (and PVS is low), these patients have a likelihood of clinical heart failure with increased intra-cardiac filling pressures and will benefit from vasodilators first, followed by diuretics therapy. When PVS values are high (and the ReDS value is low), these patients may have volume overload due to chronic kidney disease. Diuretics may be beneficial instead of heart failure-specific therapies to address systemic congestion. When patients had high ReDS values and high PVS, they would have both pulmonary and systemic congestion probably due to heart failure and renal impairment accompanying hemodynamic deterioration. Aggressive dehydration therapy using multiple therapeutic modalities would be required.

On the contrary, ReDS values and PVS were not significantly stratified by the existence of heart failure. These are not diagnostic tools. Instead, we can quantify the amount and distribution of body fluid and adjust medications by referencing their combination, irrespective of any etiologies.

4.4. Study Limitations

This study is not without limitations. It consists of a moderate sample-sized cohort collected from a single center. Our cohort included relatively more patients with chronic kidney disease compared with other studies probably due to a relatively higher age and multiple comorbidities. Our findings may not simply be adopted to other cohorts given the lack of validation thus far. Further larger-scale multi-institutional studies are warranted to validate and generalize our findings.

Given the lack of any cutoffs of PVS, we used a mean value of the healthy cohort. A high PVS above the cutoff in this study may not indicate clinically significant systemic congestion. Thus, PVS may not be a good diagnostic tool thus far. The cutoff of PVS with any clinical implications needs investigation in future studies. We proposed a therapeutic strategy by referencing the combination of a ReDS value and PVS, though prospective validation of these modalities in guiding therapy needs further investigation.

4.5. Conclusions

The combination of ReDS values and PVS was able to better classify clinical profiles often associated with either pulmonary congestion, systemic congestion, or neither. These modalities may be useful adjunctive diagnostic tools to consider when developing a therapeutic strategy.

Author Contributions: Conceptualization, T.I. (Teruhiko Imamura); Methodology, T.I. (Teruhiko Imamura); Formal analysis, T.I. (Teruhiko Imamura); Investigation, T.I. (Teruhiko Imamura), H.O., M.N. (Masaki Nakagaito), S.T., M.N. (Makiko Nakamura), R.U., H.F. and K.K. (Kota Kakeshita); Data curation, T.I. (Toshihdie Izumida) and T.I. (Teruhiko Imamura); Writing—original draft, T.I. (Teruhiko Imamura); Writing—review & editing, N.N. and K.K. (Koichiro Kinugawa); Visualization, T.I. (Teruhiko Imamura); Supervision, K.K. (Koichiro Kinugawa); Project administration, T.I. (Teruhiko Imamura). All authors have read and agreed to the published version of the manuscript.

Funding: This research received no external funding.

Institutional Review Board Statement: The study was conducted in accordance with the Declaration of Helsinki, and approved by the Committee of Ethics, University of Toyama (MTK2020007, 3 March 2021).

Informed Consent Statement: Informed consent was obtained from all subjects involved in the study.

Data Availability Statement: Data are available upon reasonable requests.

Conflicts of Interest: The authors declare no conflict of interest.

References

1. Boorsma, E.M.; Ter Maaten, J.M.; Damman, K.; Dinh, W.; Gustafsson, F.; Goldsmith, S.; Burkhoff, D.; Zannad, F.; Udelson, J.E.; Voors, A.A. Congestion in heart failure: A contemporary look at physiology, diagnosis and treatment. *Nat. Rev. Cardiol.* **2020**, *17*, 641–655. [CrossRef] [PubMed]
2. Narang, N.; Chung, B.; Nguyen, A.; Kalathiya, R.J.; Laffin, L.J.; Holzhauser, L.; Ebong, I.A.; Besser, S.A.; Imamura, T.; Smith, B.A.; et al. Discordance Between Clinical Assessment and Invasive Hemodynamics in Patients with Advanced Heart Failure. *J. Card. Fail.* **2020**, *26*, 128–135. [CrossRef] [PubMed]
3. Imamura, T.; Narang, N.; Kinugawa, K. Clinical implications of remote dielectric sensing system to estimate lung fluid levels. *J. Cardiol.* **2022**. [CrossRef] [PubMed]
4. Imamura, T.; Hori, M.; Ueno, Y.; Narang, N.; Onoda, H.; Tanaka, S.; Nakamura, M.; Kataoka, N.; Sobajima, M.; Fukuda, N.; et al. Association between Lung Fluid Levels Estimated by Remote Dielectric Sensing Values and Invasive Hemodynamic Measurements. *J. Clin. Med.* **2022**, *11*, 1208. [CrossRef] [PubMed]
5. Imamura, T.; Gonoi, W.; Hori, M.; Ueno, Y.; Narang, N.; Onoda, H.; Tanaka, S.; Nakamura, M.; Kataoka, N.; Ushijima, R.; et al. Validation of Noninvasive Remote Dielectric Sensing System to Quantify Lung Fluid Levels. *J. Clin. Med.* **2021**, *11*, 164. [CrossRef] [PubMed]
6. Amir, O.; Azzam, Z.S.; Gaspar, T.; Faranesh-Abboud, S.; Andria, N.; Burkhoff, D.; Abbo, A.; Abraham, W.T. Validation of remote dielectric sensing (ReDS) technology for quantification of lung fluid status: Comparison to high resolution chest computed tomography in patients with and without acute heart failure. *Int. J. Cardiol.* **2016**, *221*, 841–846. [CrossRef] [PubMed]
7. Tamaki, S.; Yamada, T.; Morita, T.; Furukawa, Y.; Iwasaki, Y.; Kawasaki, M.; Kikuchi, A.; Kawai, T.; Seo, M.; Abe, M.; et al. Prognostic Value of Calculated Plasma Volume Status in Patients Admitted for Acute Decompensated Heart Failure—A Prospective Comparative Study With Other Indices of Plasma Volume. *Circ. Rep.* **2019**, *1*, 361–371. [CrossRef]
8. Martens, P.; Nijst, P.; Dupont, M.; Mullens, W. The Optimal Plasma Volume Status in Heart Failure in Relation to Clinical Outcome. *J. Card. Fail.* **2019**, *25*, 240–248. [CrossRef]
9. Ling, H.Z.; Flint, J.; Damgaard, M.; Bonfils, P.K.; Cheng, A.S.; Aggarwal, S.; Velmurugan, S.; Mendonca, M.; Rashid, M.; Kang, S.; et al. Calculated plasma volume status and prognosis in chronic heart failure. *Eur. J. Heart Fail.* **2015**, *17*, 35–43. [CrossRef] [PubMed]
10. Otaki, Y.; Watanabe, T.; Konta, T.; Watanabe, M.; Asahi, K.; Yamagata, K.; Fujimoto, S.; Tsuruya, K.; Narita, I.; Kasahara, M.; et al. Impact of calculated plasma volume status on all-cause and cardiovascular mortality: 4-year nationwide community-based prospective cohort study. *PLoS ONE* **2020**, *15*, e0237601. [CrossRef] [PubMed]
11. Izumida, T.; Imamura, T.; Kinugawa, K. Remote dielectric sensing and lung ultrasound to assess pulmonary congestion. *Heart Vessel.* **2022**. [CrossRef]
12. Shimura, T.; Yamamoto, M.; Yamaguchi, R.; Adachi, Y.; Sago, M.; Tsunaki, T.; Kagase, A.; Koyama, Y.; Otsuka, T.; Yashima, F.; et al. Calculated plasma volume status and outcomes in patients undergoing transcatheter aortic valve replacement. *ESC Heart Fail.* **2021**, *8*, 1990–2001. [CrossRef] [PubMed]
13. Maznyczka, A.M.; Barakat, M.F.; Ussen, B.; Kaura, A.; Abu-Own, H.; Jouhra, F.; Jaumdally, H.; Amin-Youssef, G.; Nicou, N.; Baghai, M.; et al. Calculated plasma volume status and outcomes in patients undergoing coronary bypass graft surgery. *Heart* **2019**, *105*, 1020–1026. [CrossRef]
14. Imamura, T.; Narang, N.; Combs, P.; Siddiqi, U.; Mirzai, S.; Stonebraker, C.; Bullard, H.; Simone, P.; Jeevanandam, V. Impact of plasma volume status on mortality following left ventricular assist device implantation. *Artif. Organs.* **2021**, *45*, 587–592. [CrossRef]
15. Parmley, W.W. Pathophysiology of congestive heart failure. *Am. J. Cardiol.* **1985**, *56*, 7A–11A. [CrossRef]
16. Hung, S.C.; Lai, Y.S.; Kuo, K.L.; Tarng, D.C. Volume overload and adverse outcomes in chronic kidney disease: Clinical observational and animal studies. *J. Am. Heart. Assoc.* **2015**, *4*, e001918. [CrossRef]

Disclaimer/Publisher's Note: The statements, opinions and data contained in all publications are solely those of the individual author(s) and contributor(s) and not of MDPI and/or the editor(s). MDPI and/or the editor(s) disclaim responsibility for any injury to people or property resulting from any ideas, methods, instructions or products referred to in the content.

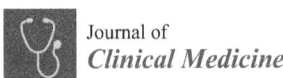

Article

Isolated Subclinical Right Ventricle Systolic Dysfunction in Patients after Liver Transplantation

Emel Celiker Guler [1,*], Mehmet Onur Omaygenc [2], Deniz Dilan Naki [2], Arzu Yazar [2], Ibrahim Oguz Karaca [2] and Esin Korkut [2]

1 Department of Cardiology, Koc University Hospital, Davutpasa Ave., No:4, Zeytinburnu, 34010 Istanbul, Turkey
2 Department of Cardiology, Istanbul Medipol University Hospital, TEM European Highway, Goztepe Exit, No:1, Bagcilar, 34214 Istanbul, Turkey
* Correspondence: emelcelikerguler@hotmail.com; Tel.: +90-532-430-8882

Abstract: Although hemodynamic alterations in end-stage liver disease (ESLD) and its association with porto-pulmonary hypertension have been well-established, the long-term effects of ESLD on RV systolic function in patients without porto-pulmonary hypertension remain disregarded. Here we aimed to assess the long-term effect of ESLD on RV function and its relationship with the use of NSBBs and clinical, laboratory and imaging parameters in end-stage liver disease. The use of NSBBs is still controversial due to concerns about reduced cardiac contractility and the possibility of increased mortality. Thirty-four liver transplant recipients were included. Demographic characteristics, laboratory and baseline echocardiography measures were obtained. Patients were recalled for transthoracic echocardiographic evaluation after transplantation. Right ventricle dysfunction was identified by having at least one value below the reference levels of RV S', or TAPSE. Isolated subclinical RV dysfunction was observed at 20.6% of the sample population. The present study demonstrates hemodynamic circulation in cirrhosis and increased preload and afterload might have long-term effects on RV function, even the lack of porto-pulmonary hypertension. These findings underline the significance of cardiac function follow-up in cirrhotic patients after transplantation. In this study, patients treated with propranolol seemed to have better RV function and less gastrointestinal bleeding. We speculated that preoperative propranolol treatment might help preserve RV function by providing RAS suppression, improving endothelial function and hyperdynamic circulation seen in ESLD. This potential protective relationship between the use of propranolol and RV function might improve mortality or graft-failure during OLT and after liver transplantation in patients with cirrhosis.

Keywords: end-stage chronic liver disease; liver transplantation; heart failure; right ventricle function; propranolol

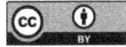

1. Introduction

End-stage liver disease (ESLD) affects the pulmonary and cardiac structure and function through several mechanisms. Although the exact mechanism is not clear yet, several hypotheses including hyperdynamic circulation, excess production and impaired clearance of vasoactive substances, portosystemic shunt and genetic predisposition are considered to have a role in this multisystemic effect [1–3]. Hyperdynamic circulation refers to increased cardiac output (CO), reduced systemic vascular resistance and splanchnic vasodilation noted in patients with cirrhosis [4,5]. High CO may lead to endothelial dysfunction due to shear wall stress. Moreover, toxic substances that bypass the liver through the portosystemic shunt may also cause direct damage to the pulmonary arteriolar endothelium [3,4,6]. These multifactorial mechanisms may result in excessive pulmonary vascular remodeling, increased pulmonary vascular pressures and pulmonary vascular resistance (PVR), and consequently, right ventricular (RV) dysfunction [7]. Although more commonly considered in the context of pulmonary hypertension, cirrhotic cardiomyopathy also induces left ventricle (LV) dysfunction and rising RV afterload owing to increased LV diastolic pressures. Severely increased RV afterload is recognized as a risk factor for mortality in liver transplant candidates. The deterioration of RV function has been demonstrated to be superior to LV dysfunction in predicting adverse clinical outcomes and mortality during orthotopic liver transplantation (OLT) [8].

Non-selective beta blockers (NSBBs) are recommended for the primary and secondary prevention of variceal bleeding in patients with cirrhosis [9–13]; their protective effect on recurrent gastrointestinal bleeding was first introduced in the literature almost 40 years ago [13]. Non-selective beta blockers reduce portal hypertension by reducing portal venous flow through splanchnic vasoconstriction. Moreover, NSBBs might decrease systemic inflammation via increased intestinal transit and reduced gut permeability [14]. Many studies have shown that NSBBs are associated with improved survival in patients with cirrhosis [15,16]; however, the use of NSBBs in ESLD is still controversial due to their harmful effects on cardiac contractility and mean arterial pressure [17,18]. However, compared to NSBBs, selective beta-1 antagonists such as atenolol and metoprolol have been shown to be less effective for the prevention of variceal bleeding [19,20]. Non-selective beta blockers decrease portal pressure by beta-2 adrenergic blockage, which causes splanchnic vasoconstriction; however, selective beta-1 antagonists have no effect on portal pressure. A prospective randomized trial assessed for the value of selective beta-1 antagonists for the long-term management of variceal bleeding showed that metoprolol was associated with a significantly higher risk of recurrent variceal bleeding compared to injection sclerotherapy [19].

Two-dimensional (2D) transthoracic echocardiography is a routine examination for the assessment of porto-pulmonary hypertension [21], RV/LV structure and function [22,23], porto-pulmonary shunt [24] and the necessity of right heart catheterization among patients with ESLD being considered for liver transplantation. The association of RV functional impairment and advanced chronic liver disease in patients with porto-pulmonary hypertension has been well-established. However, the long-term effects of ESLD and increased RV afterload in RV systolic function remain disregarded especially in cirrhotic patients without signs of porto-pulmonary hypertension. Therefore, we sought to determine whether ESLD would have long-term effects on RV function and cause subclinical RV systolic dysfunction without the clinical/echocardiographic signs of porto-pulmonary hypertension. Finally, we sought to determine the impact of non-selective beta blockers and other identifiers on RV systolic function after OLT by comparing the baseline characteristics and follow-up echocardiographic parameters.

2. Materials and Methods

2.1. Study Population

The analysis was performed on consecutive adult ESLD patients (age > 18 years) who underwent their first liver transplantation at Medipol University from June 2014 to September 2019. At our institution, echocardiography is a standard of care for all OLT candidates. Orthotopic liver transplantation candidates who had significant left heart disease, severe chronic pulmonary disease, any identified previous episode of pulmonary embolism, hepatocellular carcinoma as the etiology for transplant, <6 months between transplant and echocardiographic follow-up or the absence of critical retrospective data were excluded. Demographic and baseline clinical features at the time of surgery were noted. Preoperative laboratory work-up, estimated systolic pulmonary arterial pressure (sPAP) value at preoperative cardiology consultation and post-transplantation early hepatic and portal venous duplex ultrasound findings were recorded. Patients were recalled for follow-up echocardiographic examination.

The study was approved by the Institutional Ethics Review Committee of Medipol University (299/20 and 16 April 2020).

2.2. Echocardiography

Echocardiography was performed using a commercially available echocardiography system (Vivid 7 or E9 (General Electric-Vingmed, Horten, Norway)) and the obtained images were digitally stored in cine-loop format. The EchoPAC system was used for offline analysis (EchoPAC version 112.0.1; General Electric-Vingmed Ultrasound, Horten, Norway). The standard biplane Simpson method was used to calculate the left ventricular ejection fraction (LVEF) [13]. Pulsed-Doppler echocardiography was performed to measure peak early diastolic transmitral flow velocity (E) [13]. The early diastolic velocity of the lateral and septal aspects of the mitral annulus (E') was measured by Doppler tissue imaging and was averaged to acquire E'. The E/E' ratio was calculated by dividing the peak inflow velocity by the averaged annular velocities [23]. The maximum tricuspid regurgitant jet gradient was calculated by using the modified Bernoulli equation [14]. Systolic pulmonary arterial pressure was calculated by summating the tricuspid regurgitant gradient and right atrial pressure. Tricuspid annular plane systolic excursion (TAPSE) was measured from M-mode recordings of the lateral tricuspid annulus in the RV view [25]. Measurements of tricuspid annular systolic velocity (TAs) were obtained using tissue Doppler imaging [14].

2.3. Statistical Analysis

The data were presented as mean ± standard deviation and median (range) for continuous variables and percentage for categorical variables. Shapiro–Wilk test was used to determine whether a continuous variable followed normal distribution or not. To discriminate the patients with and without right ventricular dysfunction, Student's t and Mann–Whitney U tests were utilized for comparing the variables showing normal and non-normal distribution, respectively. The frequencies of categorical variables were distinguished by the chi-square test. Two-sided $p \leq 0.05$ was interpreted as statistically significant. Statistical analyses were carried out by using SPSS (version 17.0, SPSS Inc., Chicago, IL, USA).

3. Results

A total of 56 liver transplant recipients who had the complete baseline dataset were assessed for recruitment. Seven patients were excluded due to confounding medical conditions as described above (exclusion criteria: OLT candidates who had significant left heart disease, severe chronic pulmonary disease, any identified previous episode of pulmonary embolism, hepatocellular carcinoma as the etiology for transplant, <6 months between transplant and echocardiographic follow-up or the absence of critical retrospective data). Of the remaining 49 recipients, 15 individuals were lost to follow-up.

Ultimately, 34 patients (mean age 54.1 ± 8.7) constituted the sample population. Follow-up echocardiography was performed after a mean duration of 18 ± 6 months following OLT. At the follow-up visit, right ventricular dysfunction (RVD) was identified as the measurement of TAPSE and/or peak Doppler annular velocity (RVSm) below the reference values (<17 mm and 9.5 cm/s, respectively) suggested in the relevant position paper [13]. Isolated RV dysfunction was observed at 20.6% (n = 7) of the sample population. Patients were then grouped according to the presence of isolated RV dysfunction (Group A: liver recipients without isolated subclinical RV dysfunction and Group B: liver recipients with subclinical RV dysfunction).

Table 1 provides the baseline characteristics of the patients with isolated RV dysfunction and without RV dysfunction. The age, gender and body mass index (BMI) were similar between the two groups. The mean time between diagnosis and transplant was 5.5 ± 5.3 years and was similar in the two groups. Viral etiology hepatitis was seen in approximately half of the patients in both groups. Hepatocellular carcinoma as the etiology for transplant was excluded. Other etiologies including alcoholic liver disease and non-alcoholic fatty liver diseases were similar between the two groups. There were no statistically significant differences in the Child–Pugh score, Model for End-stage Liver Disease (MELD) score and esophageal variceal grade between the two groups; however, gastrointestinal bleeding was higher in group B (Table 1). The history of hypertension and smoking between the two groups showed no significant difference. However, the history of coronary artery disease (CAD) was higher in group B. Treatment with spironolactone, other diuretics, renin-angiotensin system blocking agents (RAS-B) and calcium channel blockers (CCB) was similar in both groups. In contrast, treatment with a non-selective beta blocker (propranolol) was higher in group A (Table 1).

Table 1. Baseline characteristics of the liver transplant recipients.

	Overall (n = 34)	RVD (−) (n = 27)	RVD (+) (n = 7)	p Value
Age, years; Mean ± SD	54.1 ± 8.7	53.6 ± 8.7	56.1 ± 9.1	0.65
Gender, female; % (n)	32.4 (11)	29.6 (8)	42.9 (3)	0.51
BMI, kg/m^2; Median (Range)	29.6 [11.5]	29.4 [11.5]	30.5 [7.4]	0.40
Diagnosis-to-transplantation time, years; Mean ± SD	5.5 ± 5.3	5.8 ± 5.5	4.6 ± 4.3	0.71
Etiology, viral; % (n)	47.1 (16)	48.1 (13)	42.9 (3)	0.80
Child–Pugh score; Mean ± SD	8.2 ± 1.6	8.3 ± 1.5	8.5 ± 2.6	0.43
MELD score; Mean ± SD	18.3 ± 6.3	19.3 ± 6.3	14.6 ± 5.1	0.06
Esophageal varices grade; Mean ± SD	1.4 ± 1.1	1.5 ± 1.1	1.3 ± 1.1	0.65
History of GI Bleeding; % (n)	17.6 (6)	11.1 (3)	42.9 (3)	**0.05**
Hypertension; % (n)	38.2 (13)	44.4 (12)	14.3 (1)	0.14
Smoking history (>20 package years); % (n)	41.2 (14)	37 (10)	57.1 (4)	0.34
Coronary artery disease; % (n)	5.9 (2)	0 (0)	28.6 (2)	**<0.01**
Propranolol use; % (n)	52.9 (18)	63 (17)	14.3 (1)	**0.02**
Spironolactone use; % (n)	61.8 (21)	63 (17)	57.1 (4)	0.78
Other diuretic use; % (n)	67.6 (23)	66.7 (18)	71.4 (5)	0.81
RAS-B use; % (n)	14.7 (5)	18.5 (5)	0 (0)	0.22
CCB use; % (n)	17.6 (6)	18.5 (5)	14.3 (1)	0.79

The choice of non-selective beta blocker was propranolol, as nadolol is non-available in Turkey. Patients who used selective beta-blocking agents due to coronary artery disease and hypertension and did not use propranolol seemed to have higher rates of isolated RV dysfunction (RVD) (Figure 1).

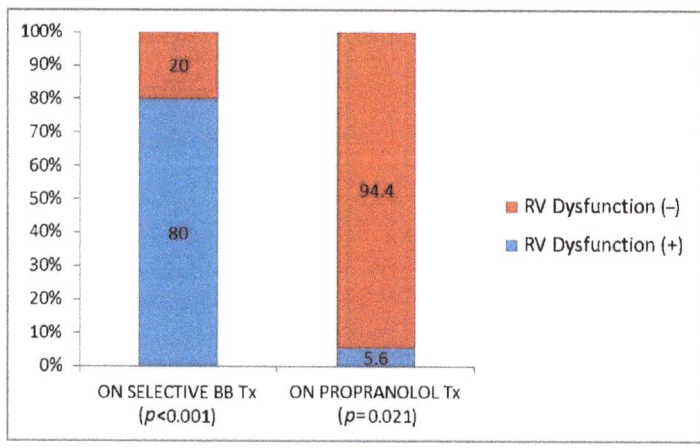

Figure 1. Relationship of non-selective beta blocker and isolated subclinical RVD.

Preoperative laboratory test variables between the two groups including estimated glomerular filtration rate (eGFR), albumin, INR, ALT, GGT, hemoglobin, platelet count, CRP and pro-BNP were similar (Table 2). In addition, preoperative hepatic and portal venous duplex US findings were similar between the two groups (Table 2).

Table 2. Preoperative laboratory test results and hepatic and portal venous duplex US findings of the liver transplant recipients.

	RVD (−) (n = 27)	RVD (+) (n = 7)	p Value
eGFR, mL/min/1.73 m^2; Median (Range)	99.7 [143.5]	99.8 [85.2]	0.93
Albumin, g/dL; Mean ± SD	3.3 ± 0.6	3.3 ± 0.6	0.97
INR, Median (Range)	1.5 [2.1]	1.5 [1]	0.93
ALT, U/L; Mean ± SD	42 ± 31.1	39.5 ± 26.7	0.87
GGT, U/L; Mean ± SD	69 ± 62.1	131 ± 119.5	0.16
Hemoglobin, g/dL; Median (Range)	10.5 [9.2]	12.6 [5]	0.24
Platelet count, ×1000/μL; Mean ± SD	87.8 ± 55.8	148.1 ± 152.9	0.59
CRP, mg/L; Mean ±SD	16.3 ± 24.5	14 ± 18.1	0.90
NT-ProBNP, pg/mL; Mean ± SD	161 ± 166.5	257.9 ± 353.8	0.30
Portal vein diameter, mm; Median (Range)	10 [7.2]	11 [3.8]	0.59
Portal vein velocity, cm/s; Mean ± SD	113.4 ± 77.2	72.3 ± 45.4	0.18
Portal vein output, mL/min; Mean ± SD	2460 ± 1787	2122 ± 1125	0.87
Hepatic vein velocity, cm/s; Mean ± SD	59.7 ± 32.4	56 ± 36	0.62

A comparison of echocardiographic parameters in the two groups is shown in Table 3. In both groups, preoperative and follow-up sPAP values were within the normal range. There was no statistical difference between the two groups in LV Ejection Fraction (LVEF), E/E', LV/RV ratio and RA area.

Table 3. Preoperative and follow-up echocardiography parameters in liver transplant recipients.

	RVD (−) (n = 27)	RVD (+) (n = 7)	p Value
Initial estimated sPAP, mmHg; Mean ± SD	29.6 ± 6	28.3 ± 2.2	0.68
Follow-up estimated sPAP, mmHg; Mean ± SD	28 ± 7.5	27.6 ± 7	0.87
LVEF, %; Mean ± SD	64 ± 3.3	63.3 ± 2.6	0.29
E/E'; Mean ± SD	7.2 ± 1.9	7 ± 2.2	0.84
RV:LV ratio; Median (Range)	0.75 [0.28]	0.77 [0.35]	0.36
RA area, cm^2; Median (Range)	12.5 [11.6]	14.4 [7]	0.45

4. Discussion

In this study, we demonstrated that ESLD has long-term effects on RV function. To the best of our knowledge, this is the first study describing the term "Isolated subclinical right ventricular dysfunction" after orthotopic liver Tx. It is noted that increased preload and afterload in ESLD have an impact on RV function even in the absence of porto-pulmonary hypertension. This study underlines the importance of the long-term follow-up of cardiac functions in patients with cirrhosis. In addition, we also noted that preoperative treatment with propranolol might help preserve RV function. There might be a potential protective relationship between the use of propranolol and RV function in patients with cirrhosis. This finding can be explained by the beneficial effects of PPL in endothelial function, RAS suppression and hyperdynamic circulation that might promote RV function during long-term follow-up in patients with ESLD. Moreover, the patients treated with non-selective beta-blockers had less gastrointestinal bleeding than those who did not use propranolol. This finding agrees with the previous studies, as propranolol is considered effective in the primary and secondary prevention of variceal bleeding.

The clinical importance of subclinical RV dysfunction and its association with adverse clinical outcomes has been investigated in different clinical scenarios [26–31]. In ESLD, RV afterload and preload are affected due to several hemodynamical consequences of advanced liver disease including hyperdynamic circulation, increased pulmonary vascular resistance and increased LV diastolic pressure with a subsequent increase in pulmonary wedge pressure [3–7]. Given the sensitivity of RV to dynamic alterations in preload and afterload, these multifactorial mechanisms in advanced liver disease can be a concern in the development of RV overload and dysfunction. Demirtas Inci et al. compared the global LV and RV functions of forty liver transplant candidates with ESLD and twenty-six healthy individuals [32]. The 2D speckle tracking method was preferred for the mean longitudinal, circumferential and radial strain measurements. They noted that LV mean radial/longitudinal and RV mean longitudinal strain were significantly lower in the patient group. The study concluded that the deterioration of longitudinal and radial deformation is a sign of the subclinical impairment of global LV and RV systolic functions in liver transplant candidates [32].

Other studies have evaluated RV function in ESLD patients while awaiting and during transplants [22,33,34]. A retrospective study compared TAPSE and TAs between a group of ESLD patients being considered for OLT and patients without the liver disease [22]. All patients included in the study had normal LV systolic function and normal pulmonary artery systolic pressures [22]. They found that TAPSE and TAs values were significantly higher in patients with ESLD awaiting liver transplantation [34]. The authors suggested the differences in echocardiographic indices of RV systolic function led to a hyperdynamic circulatory state in ESLD patients [34]. A limitation of this study is the unknown long-term impact of this compensatory mechanism on RV function following transplantation. Right ventricle function during classic OLT has also been investigated [34]. Xu et al. examined RVEF using a modified pulmonary artery catheter during OLT in a study of thirty patients [34]. Baseline RVEF was found to be lower than the normal value. In addition, Xu et al. noted that RVEF was impaired during the anhepatic and early reperfusion stages. The authors highlighted that the RV function plays a crucial role in maintaining stable hemodynamics and close monitoring of the RV function is essential [34]. Moreover, a study has shown that right heart-associated hemodynamic factors were associated with patient survival after liver transplantation or graft failure [35]. Even though no association between the time-weighted LV stroke work index and PVR for one-year mortality was demonstrated, the time-weighted mean RV stroke work index was found significantly related with one-year all-cause mortality. The study advised that the intraoperative RV stroke work index might be a prognostic marker for mortality after liver transplantation [35]. In our study, patients treated with NSBBs had significantly less RV systolic dysfunction, which might be associated with good outcome in this population both during transplantation and follow-up.

Non-selective beta blocker agents, mostly propranolol (PPL), are used for the primary and secondary prophylaxis of acute and chronic gastrointestinal (GI) bleeding caused by esophageal varices in patients with cirrhosis. Carvedilol, nebivolol and nadolol are alternative agents [36,37]. Propranolol decreases portal hypertension and portal blood flow by reducing CO and splanchnic vasoconstriction [38,39]. In our study, the preferred non-selective beta blocker was propranolol. Indeed, carvedilol would be the preferred B blocker agent because, in recent years, several studies demonstrated that it was better in long-term HVPG reduction due to its anti-alpha-adrenergic activity and ability to improve the release of nitric oxide. Furthermore, a recent study demonstrated that patients treated with carvedilol had better adherence to therapy and outcome than propranolol [40]. However, most of these findings were obtained after this study was designed. Additionally, nadolol was not preferred as it is non-available in our country. Our study found that the patients treated with propranolol had less gastrointestinal bleeding.

Besides the beneficial effects of propranolol in reducing hepatic vein pressure gradient (HVPG), it has been reported in some studies that propranolol might alleviate inflammatory response, reduce bacterial translocation, improve endothelial function, reduce the angiotensin levels in the portal vein and peripheral vasculature [41–44]. A prospective controlled study investigated PPL's vascular function and impact using venous occlusion plethysmography [43]. The authors demonstrated the gradual deterioration of endothelial function in cirrhotic patients not treated with PPL; nevertheless, there was an improvement in Child–Pugh score in patients treated with PPL [43]. These findings also supported another study that included 38 cirrhotic outpatients with ascites, divided into two groups according to use or not of PPL [41]. They demonstrated that PPL might protect the endothelium from inflammatory exhaustion and improve hemodynamic status [41]. Furthermore, Vilas-Boas et al. found that treatment with PPL reduced the Renin–Angiotensin System (RAS) mediators and could change the prognosis of patients with hyperdynamic circulation [43]. In the present study, we demonstrated that the patients treated with PPL had significantly lower rates of isolated RV dysfunction compared to those not treated with PPL. The reduced RAS activation and decreased hyperdynamic circulation, in addition to a less inflammatory response with PPL, might be protective of RV function during long-term follow-up.

On the contrary, a study investigated increased mortality with NSBBs in patients with refractory ascites and cirrhosis [17]. This single-center study evaluated 1-year survival at 19% in patients treated with propranolol; however, 1 year survival of 64% in patients not treated with propranolol suggested that the use of propranolol in patients with cirrhosis and refractory ascites was associated with poor survival [17]. Furthermore, 'the window therapy hypotheses' were proposed by Krag et al., where NSBBs would be used in the early stages without severe varices and should be stopped in end-stage cirrhosis because they would reduce cardiac contractility, worsening systemic perfusion and prognosis [18]. In advanced cirrhosis, compensatory mechanisms including up-regulation of the sympathetic nervous system [45,46] and renin-angiotensin-aldosterone system [47,48] exist to maintain proper cardiac output and organ perfusion; however, these compensatory mechanisms fail as cirrhosis progresses. In this advanced stage, the maintenance of cardiac output and mean arterial pressure is essential to improve survival. However, recent studies and the BANEVO VII guidelines recommended the use of NSBBs in all patients with clinically significant portal hypertension [49]. The PREDESCI trial, a multicenter, double-blind and first randomized controlled trial, showed that long-term treatment with NSBBs reduces clinical decompensation or cirrhosis-related mortality by reducing the rates of ascites. The study suggested that the long-term treatment of cirrhotic patients with NSBBs might prevent progression to clinical decompensation or death [40].

Some limitations should be acknowledged, such as the single-center nature of the study, the selection biases of a retrospective study and sample size. Moreover, only 2D echocardiographic parameters were assessed for the evaluation of RV function. Strain imaging and novel 3-dimensional echocardiography are preferred to support the present study's findings.

5. Conclusions

To the best of our knowledge, this is the first study describing the term "Isolated subclinical right ventricular dysfunction" after orthotopic liver Tx. We hypothesized that the impact of propranolol on RAS suppression, hemodynamic circulation and endothelial function might help preserve RV function during long-term follow-up via a more prominent reduction in hepatic venous gradient at the preoperative stage. This potential protective relationship between the use of propranolol and RV function in patients with cirrhosis might improve mortality or graft-failure after liver transplantation. However, future studies with more robust designs are necessary to verify this association and the hypothesis should be supported by evidence obtained via biochemical work-up.

Author Contributions: Conceptualization, M.O.O., D.D.N., I.O.K. and E.K.; methodology, E.C.G., M.O.O., I.O.K. and E.K.; formal analysis E.C.G. and M.O.O.; investigation, E.C.G., M.O.O. and D.D.N.; project administration M.O.O.; resources, A.Y. and D.D.N.; data curation, M.O.O., D.D.N., A.Y. and I.O.K.; writing—original draft preparation, E.C.G. and M.O.O.; writing—review and editing, supervision E.C.G.; visualization, E.C.G. and M.O.O. All authors have read and agreed to the published version of the manuscript.

Funding: This research received no external funding.

Institutional Review Board Statement: The study was conducted in accordance with the Declaration of Helsinki and approved by the Institutional Ethics Committee of Medipol University (299/20 and 16 April 2020).

Informed Consent Statement: Informed consent was obtained from all subjects involved in the study.

Data Availability Statement: The data presented in this study are available on request from the corresponding author. The data are not publicly available due to privacy restrictions.

Conflicts of Interest: The authors declare no conflict of interest.

References

1. Battista, S.; Bar, F.; Mengozzi, G.; Zanon, E.; Grosso, M.; Molino, G. Hyperdynamic circulation in patients with cirrhosis: Direct measurement of nitric oxide levels in hepatic and portal veins. *J. Hepatol.* **1997**, *26*, 75–80. [CrossRef]
2. Savale, L.; Watherald, J.; Sitbon, O. Portopulmonary Hypertension. *Semin. Respir. Crit. Care Med.* **2017**, *38*, 651–661. [PubMed]
3. Liberal, R.; Grant, C.R.; Baptista, R.; Macedo, G. Porto-pulmonary hypertension: A comprehensive review. *Clin. Res. Hepatol. Gastroenterol.* **2015**, *39*, 157–167. [CrossRef] [PubMed]
4. Herve, P.; Lebrec, D.; Brenot, F.; Simonneau, G.; Humbert, M.; Sitbon, O.; Duroux, P. Pulmonary vascular disorders in portal hypertension. *Eur. Respir. J.* **1998**, *11*, 1153–1166. [CrossRef]
5. Rodríguez-Vilarrupla, A.; Fernández, M.; Bosch, J.; García-Pagán, J.C. Current concepts on the pathophysiology of portal hypertension. *Ann. Hepatol.* **2007**, *6*, 28–36. [CrossRef] [PubMed]
6. Herve, P.; Le Pavec, J.; Sztrymf, B.; Decante, B.; Savale, L.; Sitbon, O. Pulmonary vascular abnormalities in cirrhosis. *Best Pract. Res. Clin. Gastroenterol.* **2007**, *21*, 141–159. [CrossRef] [PubMed]
7. Wong, F.; Liu, P.; Lilly, L.; Bomzon, A.; Blendis, L. Role of cardiac structural and functional abnormalities in the pathogenesis of hyperdynamic circulation and renal sodium retention in cirrhosis. *Clin. Sci.* **1999**, *97*, 259–267. [CrossRef]
8. Kia, L.; Shah, S.J.; Wang, E.; Sharma, D.; Selvaraj, S.; Medina, C.; Cahan, J.; Mahon, H.; Levitsky, J. Role of pretransplant echocardiographic evaluation in predicting outcomes following liver transplantation. *Am. J. Transplant.* **2013**, *13*, 2395–2401. [CrossRef]
9. Jakab, S.S.; Garcia-Tsao, G. Evaluation and management of esophageal and gastric varices in patients with cirrhosis. *Clin. Liver. Dis.* **2020**, *24*, 335–350. [CrossRef]
10. Poynard, T.; Cales, P.; Pasta, L.; Ideo, G.; Pascal, J.P.; Pagliaro, L.; Lebrec, D.; Franco—Italian Multicenter Study Group. Beta-adrenergic-antagonist drugs in the prevention of gastrointestinal bleeding in patients with cirrhosis and esophageal varices: An analysis of data and prognostic factors in 589 patients from four randomized clinical trials. *N. Engl. J. Med.* **1991**, *324*, 1532–1538.
11. Pascal, J.P.; Cales, P. Propranolol in the prevention of first upper gastrointestinal tract hemorrhage in patients with cirrhosis of the liver and esophageal varices. *N. Engl. J. Med.* **1987**, *317*, 856–861. [CrossRef] [PubMed]
12. Garcia-Tsao, G.; Bosch, J. Management of varices and variceal hemorrhage in cirrhosis. *N. Engl. J. Med.* **2010**, *362*, 823–832. [CrossRef] [PubMed]
13. Lebrec, D.; Corbic, M.; Nouel, O.; Benhamou, J.P. Propranolol—A medical treatment for portal hypertension? *Lancet* **1980**, *316*, 180–182. [CrossRef] [PubMed]
14. Senzolo, M.; Cholongitas, E.; Burra, P.; Leandro, G.; Thalheimer, U.; Patch, D.; Burroughs, A.K. β-Blockers protect against spontaneous bacterial peritonitis in cirrhotic patients: A meta-analysis. *Liver Int.* **2009**, *29*, 1189–1193. [CrossRef] [PubMed]
15. Lo, G.-H.; Chen, W.-C.; Lin, C.-K.; Tsai, W.-L.; Chan, H.-H.; Chen, T.-A.; Yu, H.-C.; Hsu, P.-I.; Lai, K.-H. Improved survival in patients receiving medical therapy as compared with banding ligation for the prevention of esophageal variceal rebleeding. *Hepatology* **2008**, *48*, 580–587. [CrossRef]
16. Bhutta, A.Q.; Garcia-Tsao, G.; Reddy, K.R.; Tandon, P.; Wong, F.; O'Leary, J.G.; Acharya, C.; Banerjee, D.; Abraldes, J.G.; Jones, T.M.; et al. Beta-blockers in hospitalised patients with cirrhosis and ascites: Mortality and factors determining discontinuation and reinitiation. *Aliment. Pharmacol. Ther.* **2018**, *47*, 78–85. [CrossRef] [PubMed]
17. Sersté, T.; Melot, C.; Francoz, C.; Durand, F.; Rautou, P.E.; Valla, D.; Moreau, R.; Lebrec, D. Deleterious effects of beta-blockers on survival in patients with cirrhosis and refractory ascites. *Hepatology* **2010**, *52*, 1017–1022. [CrossRef]
18. Krag, A.; Wiest, R.; Albillos, A.; Gluud, L.L. The window hypothesis: Haemodynamic and non-haemodynamic effects of β-blockers improve survival of patients with cirrhosis during a window in the disease. *Gut* **2012**, *61*, 967–969. [CrossRef]

19. Hillon, P.; Lebrec, D.; Muńoz, C.; Jungers, M.; Goldfarb, G.; Benhamou, J.P. Comparison of the effects of a cardioselective and a nonselective bblocker on portal hypertension in patients with cirrhosis. *Hepatology* **1982**, *2*, 528–531. [CrossRef]
20. Westaby, D.; Melia, W.M.; Macdougall, B.R.; Hegarty, J.E.; Gimson, A.E.; Williams, R. B1 selective adrenoreceptor blockade for the long-term management of variceal bleeding. A prospective randomised trial to compare oral metoprolol with injection sclerotherapy in cirrhosis. *Gut* **1985**, *26*, 421–425. [CrossRef]
21. Torregrosa, M.; Genesca, J.; Gonzalez, A.; Evangelista, A.; Mora, A.; Margarit, C.; Esteban, R.; Guardia, J. Role of Doppler echocardiography in the assessment of porto-pulmonary hypertension in liver transplantation candidates. *J. Hepatol.* **2005**, *42*, 68–74. [CrossRef] [PubMed]
22. López-Candales, A.; Menendez, F.L.; Shah, S.A.; Friedrich, A. Measures of right ventricular systolic function in end stage liver disease patients awaiting transplant. *Int. J. Cardiol.* **2014**, *171*, 277–278. [CrossRef] [PubMed]
23. Chen, Y.; Chan, A.C.; Chan, S.C.; Chok, S.H.; Sharr, W.; Fung, J.; Liu, J.H.; Zhen, Z.; Sin, W.C.; Lo, C.M.; et al. A detailed evaluation of cardiac function in cirrhotic patients and its alteration with or without liver transplantation. *J. Cardiol.* **2016**, *67*, 140–146. [CrossRef] [PubMed]
24. Sussman, N.L.; Kochar, R.; Fallon, M.B. Pulmonary complications in cirrhosis. *Curr. Opin. Organ. Transplant.* **2011**, *16*, 281–288. [CrossRef]
25. Lang, R.M.; Badano, L.P.; Mor-Avi, V.; Afilalo, J.; Armstrong, A.; Ernande, L.; Flachskampf, F.A.; Foster, E.; Goldstein, S.A.; Kuznetsova, T.; et al. Recommendations for cardiac chamber quantification by echocardiography in adults: An update from the American Society of Echocardiography and the European Association of Cardiovascular Imaging. *J. Am. Soc. Echocardiogr.* **2015**, *28*, 1–39.e14. [CrossRef]
26. Rudski, L.G.; Lai, W.W.; Afilalo, J.; Hua, L.; Handschumacher, M.D.; Chandrasekaran, K.; Solomon, S.D.; Louie, E.K.; Schiller, N.B. Guidelines for the echocardiographic assessment of the right heart in adults: A report from the American Society of Echocardiography endorsed by the European Association of Echocardiography, a registered branch of the European Society of Cardiology, and the Canadian Society of Echocardiography. *J. Am. Soc. Echocardiogr.* **2010**, *23*, 685–713.
27. Haddad, F.; Doyle, R.; Murphy, D.J.; Hunt, S.A. Right ventricular function in cardiovascular disease, partII: Pathophysiology, clinical importance, and management of right ventricular failure. *Circulation* **2008**, *117*, 1717–1731. [CrossRef]
28. Voelkel, N.F.; Quaife, R.A.; Leinwand, L.A.; Barst, R.J.; McGoon, M.D.; Meldrum, D.R.; Dupuis, J.; Long, C.S.; Rubin, L.J.; Smart, F.W.; et al. Right ventricular function and failure: Report of a National Heart, Lung, and Blood Institute working group on cellular and molecular mechanisms of right heart failure. *Circulation* **2006**, *114*, 1883–1891. [CrossRef]
29. Matthews, J.C.; Dardas, T.F.; Dorsch, M.P.; Aaronson, K.D. Right-sided heart failure: Diagnosis and treatment strategies. *Curr. Treat. Opt. Cardiovasc. Med.* **2008**, *10*, 329–341. [CrossRef]
30. Hernandez-Suarez, D.; López-Candales, A. Subclinical Right Ventricular Dysfunction in Patients with Severe Aortic Stenosis: A Retrospective Case Series. *Cardiol. Ther.* **2017**, *6*, 151–155. [CrossRef]
31. Towheed, A.; Sabbagh, E.; Gupta, R.; Assiri, S.; Chowdhury, M.A.; Moukarbel, G.V.; Khuder, S.A.; Schwann, T.A.; Bonnell, M.R.; Cooper, C.J.; et al. Right ventricular dysfunction and short-term outcomes following left-sided valvular surgery: An echocardiographic study. *J. Am. Heart Assoc.* **2021**, *10*, 1–13. [CrossRef] [PubMed]
32. Demirtaş Inci, S.; Sade, L.E.; Altın, C.; Pirat, B.; Erken Pamukcu, H.; Yılmaz, S.; Müderrisoğlu, H. Subclinical myocardial dysfunction in liver transplant candidates determined using speckle tracking imaging. *Turk. Kardiyol. Dern. Ars.* **2019**, *47*, 638–645. [CrossRef]
33. Acosta, F.; Sansano, T.; Palenciano, C.G.; Roqués, V.; Clavel, N.; González, P.; Robles, R.; Bueno, F.S.; Ramirez, P.; Parrilla, P. Relationship Between Cardiovascular State and Degree of Hepatic Dysfunction in Patients Treated with Liver Transplantation. *Transplant Proc.* **2016**, *8*, 231–262. [CrossRef]
34. Xu, H.; Li, W.; Xu, Z.; Shi, X. Evaluation of the right ventricular ejection fraction during classic orthotopic liver transplantation without venovenous bypass. *Clin. Transplant.* **2012**, *26*, E485–E491. [CrossRef] [PubMed]
35. Jeong, Y.H.; Yang, S.-M.; Cho, H.; Ju, J.-W.; Jang, H.S.; Lee, H.-J.; Kim, W.H. The Prognostic Role of Right Ventricular Stroke Work Index during Liver Transplantation. *J. Clin. Med.* **2021**, *10*, 4022. [CrossRef] [PubMed]
36. Gjeorgjievski, M.; Cappell, M.S. Portal hypertensive gastropathy: A systematic review of the pathophysiology, clinical presentation, natural history and therapy. *World J. Hepatol.* **2016**, *8*, 231–262. [CrossRef]
37. Li, T.; Ke, W.; Sun, P.; Chen, X.; Belgaumkar, A.; Huang, Y.; Xian, W.; Li, J.; Zheng, Q. Carvedilol for portal hypertension in cirrhosis: Systematic review with meta-analysis. *BMJ Open.* **2016**, *6*, e010902. [CrossRef]
38. La Mura, V.; Abraldes, J.G.; Raffa, S.; Retto, O.; Berzigotti, A.; García-Pagán, J.C.; Bosch, J. Prognostic value of acute hemodynamic response to i.v. propranolol in patients with cirrhosis and portal hypertension. *J. Hepatol.* **2009**, *51*, 279–287. [CrossRef]
39. Garcia-Tsao, G.; Sanyal, A.J.; Grace, N.D.; Carey, W.; Practice Guidelines Committee of the American Association for the Study of Liver Diseases; Practice Parameters Committee of the American College of Gastroenterology. Prevention and management of gastroesophageal varices and variceal hemorrhage in cirrhosis. *Hepatology* **2007**, *46*, 922–938. [CrossRef]
40. Villanueva, C.; Albillos, A.; Genescà, J.; Garcia-Pagan, J.C.; Calleja, J.L.; Aracil, C.; Bañares, R.; Morillas, R.M.; Poca, M.; Peñas, B.; et al. β blockers to prevent decompensation of cirrhosis in patients with clinically significant portal hypertension (PREDESCI): A randomised, double-blind, placebo-controlled, multicentre trial. *Lancet* **2019**, *393*, 1597–1608. [CrossRef]

41. Brito-Azevedo, A.; Perez, R.M.; Coelho, H.S.; Fernandes, E.S.; Castiglione, R.C.; Villela-Nogueira, C.A.; Bouskela, E. The anti-inflammatory role of propranolol in cirrhosis: Preventing the inflammatory exhaustion? *J. Hepatol.* **2017**, *66*, 240–241. [CrossRef]
42. Reiberger, T.; Ferlitsch, A.; Payer, B.A.; Mandorfer, M.; Heinisch, B.B.; Hayden, H.; Lammert, F.; Trauner, M.; Peck-Radosavljevic, M.; Vogelsang, H. Non-selective betablocker therapy decreases intestinal permeability and serum levels of LBP and IL-6 in patients with cirrhosis. *J. Hepatol.* **2013**, *58*, 911–921. [CrossRef] [PubMed]
43. Brito-Azevedo, A.; Perez Rde, M.; Coelho, H.S.; Fernandes Ede, S.; Castiglione, R.C.; Villela-Nogueira, C.A.; Bouskela, E. Propranolol improves endothelial dysfunction in advanced cirrhosis: The 'endothelial exhaustion' hypothesis. *Gut* **2016**, *65*, 1391–1392. [CrossRef] [PubMed]
44. Vilas-Boas, W.W.; Ribeiro-Oliveira, A., Jr.; Ribeiro Rda, C.; Vieira, R.L.; Almeida, J.; Nadu, A.P.; Simões e Silva, A.C.; Santos, R.A. Effect of propranolol on the splanchnic and peripheral renin angiotensin system in cirrhotic patients. *World J. Gastroenterol.* **2008**, *14*, 6824–6830. [CrossRef] [PubMed]
45. Willett, I.; Esler, M.; Burke, F.; Leonard, P.; Dudley, F. Total and renal sympathetic nervous system activity in alcoholic cirrhosis. *J. Hepatol.* **1985**, *1*, 639–648. [CrossRef]
46. Murray, J.F.; Dawson, A.M.; Sherlock, S. Circulatory changes in chronic liverdisease. *Am. J. Med.* **1958**, *24*, 358–367. [CrossRef] [PubMed]
47. Rosoff, L., Jr.; Zia, P.; Reynolds, T.; Horton, R. Studies of renin and aldosterone in cirrhotic patients with ascites. *Gastroenterology* **1975**, *69*, 698–705. [CrossRef]
48. Rosoff, L., Jr.; Williams, J.; Moult, P.; Williams, H.; Sherlock, S. Renal hemodynamics, and the renin–angiotensin system in cirrhosis: Relationship to sodium retention. *Dig. Dis. Sci.* **1979**, *24*, 25–32. [CrossRef]
49. de Franchis, R.; Bosch, J.; Garcia-Tsao, G.; Reiberger, T.; Ripoll, C.; Baveno VII Faculty. Baveno VII-Renewing consensus in portal hypertension. *J. Hepatol.* **2022**, *76*, 959–974. [CrossRef]

Disclaimer/Publisher's Note: The statements, opinions and data contained in all publications are solely those of the individual author(s) and contributor(s) and not of MDPI and/or the editor(s). MDPI and/or the editor(s) disclaim responsibility for any injury to people or property resulting from any ideas, methods, instructions or products referred to in the content.

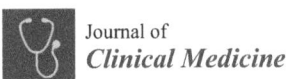

Article

sST2 and Heart Failure—Clinical Utility and Prognosis

Magdalena Dudek [1,2,*], Marta Kałużna-Oleksy [1,2], Jacek Migaj [1,2], Filip Sawczak [1,2], Helena Krysztofiak [3], Maciej Lesiak [1,2] and Ewa Straburzyńska-Migaj [1,2]

[1] 1st Department of Cardiology, Poznań University of Medical Sciences, 61-848 Poznań, Poland
[2] Heliodor Swiecicki Clinical Hospital in Poznan, 60-355 Poznań, Poland
[3] Department of Cardiology, University Hospital in Opole, 45-401 Opole, Poland
[*] Correspondence: magdamroz8@gmail.com

Abstract: New parameters and markers are constantly being sought to help better assess patients with heart failure (HF). ST2 protein has gained interest as a potential biomarker in cardiovascular disease. It is known that the IL-33/ST2L system belongs to the cardioprotective pathway, which prevents the fibrosis, hypertrophy, and apoptosis of cardiomyocytes and also inhibits the inflammatory response. Soluble ST2 (sST2) is involved in the immune response and secreted in response to the mechanical overload of the myocardium, thus providing information on the processes of myocardial remodeling and fibrosis. A total of 110 hospitalized patients diagnosed with heart failure with reduced ejection fraction (HFrEF) were included in the study. Clinical and biochemical parameters were studied. During the follow-up, 30.9% patients died and 57.3% patients reached the composite endpoint. Using ROC curves, the reference cut-off point for sST2 was determined to be 45.818 pg/mL for all-cause deaths. Significantly higher concentrations of inflammatory parameters and natriuretic peptides were found in the group of patients with higher sST2 concentrations. sST2 protein is an independent risk factor for all-cause deaths of patients with HFrEF.

Keywords: sST2; heart failure; biomarker; HFrEF

1. Introduction

Chronic heart failure (CHF) is a serious clinical syndrome and a cause of medical and social problems in industrialized countries [1]. HF is one of the major global health problems. It is estimated that in developed countries, HF affects up to 2% of the adult population [2]. A continuous increase in the prevalence of HF has been suggested, while the current prevalence is estimated to be approximately 26 million patients [3]. It should be noted that CHF significantly reduces patients' quality of life, is an important cause of hospitalization, and the 5-year mortality rate is higher than that caused by many common malignancies [4–6]. Despite significant progress in understanding the mechanisms of HF development, the implementation of prophylaxis, and the introduction of new therapeutic methods, the prognosis of this group of patients is still poor. New parameters and markers are constantly being sought to help better assess patients with HF, which could translate into better care and an improved prognosis.

ST2 (suppression of tumorigenicity 2) protein has gained interest as a potential biomarker in cardiovascular disease. It is known that the IL-33/ST2L system belongs to the cardioprotective pathway, which prevents the fibrosis, hypertrophy, and apoptosis of cardiomyocytes and also inhibits the inflammatory response. ST2 is involved in the immune response and is secreted in response to the mechanical overload of the myocardium, thus providing information on the processes of remodeling and fibrosis [7]. Soluble ST2 (sST2) acts as a decoy receptor directly bound to IL-33 and reverses the beneficial effects of the IL-33/ST2 system [8]. Plasma levels of sST2 in the general population have been found to be associated with systolic blood pressure (SBP) values [8]. Patients with HF with

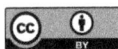

preserved ejection fraction and hypertension had higher plasma levels of sST2 compared to patients without left ventricular hypertrophy.

In recent years, studies on the use of sST2 protein as a biomarker in acute and chronic HF have been published. In recent years, studies have been published on the usefulness of the sST2 as a biomarker in acute [9] and chronic decompensated HF [10].

We aimed to assess the influence of sST2 concentration on the prognosis of patients with chronic HF.

2. Materials and Methods

2.1. Study Population

This study included patients with heart failure with reduced ejection fraction (HFrEF) who were hospitalized for the evaluation of CHF in the 1st Department of Cardiology at Poznan University of Medical Sciences in 2016–2017. The inclusion criteria were: having a left ventricle ejection fraction (LVEF) ≤45%, age ≥ 18 years, a stable period of illness (no hospitalization or need to administer intravenous diuretics due to exacerbation/decompensation of HF in the last 4 weeks), having undergone optimal pharmacological treatment according to the European Society of Cardiology 2016 Guidelines for Heart Failure [11], and having signed the informed consent form.

The study was conducted according to the guidelines of the Declaration of Helsinki, and the Ethics Committee of Poznan University of Medical Sciences approved it (No. 378/19).

2.2. Analyzed Parameters

Clinical findings were collected, including age, gender, comorbidities, prescribed medications, HF etiology, New York Heart Association (NYHA) functional class, echocardiography assessment results, and cardiopulmonary exercise test results (CPET). We analyzed complete blood count and other laboratory parameters: sST2, N-terminal pro B-type natriuretic peptide (NT-proBNP), creatinine, aspartate aminotransferase (AST), alanine aminotransferase (ALT), electrolytes (sodium and potassium), creatinine, and high-sensitivity C-reactive protein (hsCRP). sST2 concentrations from peripheral blood were calculated via the ELISA method using The Presage® ST2 Assay (Critical Diagnostics, San Diego, CA, USA) [12].

The left ventricular ejection fraction was calculated using echocardiographic Simpson's method in accordance with the ESC guidelines [13]. Breathing gas analysis was performed using the Vmax29 Sensor Medics measurement module. Patients performed a symptom-limited maximal exercise test on a treadmill according to the RAMP protocol (the load increment when inclination and treadmill travel parameters were changed was 0.5 MET/min) or according to the Bruce protocol modified for HF. Follow-up data were obtained from electronic medical records or phone conversations with patients or their family members. If follow-up data were not obtainable using either previously mentioned methods, we used National Health Fund registry data. All patients were followed up at the outpatient clinic at 3 months, and then every 6 months after enrollment in the study. During the follow-up evaluation, the primary endpoint (all-cause death) was checked.

2.3. Statistical Analysis

Statistical analysis was performed using the STATISTICA 13 program by StatSoft, owned by Tibco Software Inc. (Palo Alto, CA, USA) Continuous variables are presented as mean ± standard deviation (SD) or median (lowest quartile–highest quartile), depending on the presence of normal distribution. Categorical variables are presented as numbers (%).

Subjects were divided into two groups based on their survival. In addition, the optimal cut-off point for sST2 protein concentration to predict death from any cause was determined by analysis of the ROC curve, and participants were also grouped based on this cut-off point. Analysis of the time to death in the study groups was carried out using Kaplan–Meier analysis. The statistical significance threshold for all other tests was set at $p < 0.05$.

3. Results

Study Population

We enrolled 110 patients; 90% were men. The mean age was 53.1 ± 11.4 years, and the mean BMI was 28.2 ± 4.5 kg/m². The most common comorbidities were arterial hypertension (44.6%), diabetes mellitus (25.5%), chronic obstructive pulmonary disease (12.7%), and atrial fibrillation (16.4%). The median LVEF was 23.3 ± 7.9%. In the study population, 54 patients presented with NYHA classes III and IV (49%), and 56 patients presented with NYHA classes I and II (50.8%). At the time of inclusion in the study, most of the patients were given an optimal treatment for HFrEF. The baseline characteristics are presented in Table 1.

Table 1. Baseline characteristics of the studied group.

Parameter	Value ($n = 110$)
Age (years)	53.1 ± 11.4
Men	99 (90%)
BMI (kg/m²)	28.2 ± 4.5
SBP (mmHg)	108.0 ± 15.0
DBP (mmHg)	70.0 ± 9.0
LVEF (%)	23.3 ± 7.9
Duration of HF (months)	95.0 ± 86.0
Etiology of HF—CAD	56 (51%)
Etiology of HF—DCM	51 (46%)
NYHA class	2.4 ± 0.6
ICD	61 (56%)
CRT-D	29 (26%)
Comorbidities	
AF	18 (16.4%)
Arterial hypertension	49 (44.6%)
Diabetes mellitus type II	28 (25.5%)
Thyroid disease	21 (19.1%)
COPD	14 (12.7%)
Smoking at admission	14 (12.7%)
Smoking history	60 (54.6%)
Biochemical parameters	
sST2 (ng/mL)	45.5 ± 40.8
WBC (10^9/L)	7.6 ± 2.0
RBC (10^{12}/L)	4.8 ± 0.5
HGB (mmol/L)	8.9 ± 0.8
RDW (%)	15.2 ± 4.2
PLT (10^9/L)	201.9 ± 52.8

Table 1. *Cont.*

Parameter	Value (*n* = 110)
ESR (mm/h)	9.5 ± 10.2
CRP (mg/L)	4.5 ± 7.9
Na$^+$ (mmol/L)	139.3 ± 2.7
K$^+$ (mmol/L)	4.4 ± 2.0
Creatinine (umol/L)	103.0 ± 24.1
Fasting glucose (mmol/L)	6.5 ± 2.4
NT-proBNP (pg/mL)	2257.9 ± 3797.3
TSH (uIU/mL)	2.0 ± 1.7
CPET parameters	
Peak VO$_2$ (ml/kg/min)	17.4 ± 5.2
Peak VO$_2$ (L/min)	1.5 ± 0.5
Peak VO$_2$ (%)	54.3 ± 16.1
VE/VCO$_2$ slope	33 ± 7.5
PETCO$_2$ (mmHg)	33 ± 6.2
Medications	
Beta-blocker	108 (98.2%)
ACE-I/ARB	91 (82.7%)
ARNI	11 (10%)
MRA	96 (87.3%)
Loop diuretic	99 (90%)

BMI—body mass index; SBP—systolic blood pressure; DBP—diastolic blood pressure; NYHA—New York Heart Association; HF—heart failure; CAD—coronary artery disease; DCM—dilated cardiomyopathy; ICD—implantable cardioverter-defibrillator; CRT-D—cardiac resynchronization therapy defibrillator; AF—atrial fibrillation; COPD—chronic obstructive pulmonary disease; WBC—white blood cells; RBC—red blood cells; HGB—hemoglobin; RDW—red blood cell distribution width; PLT—platelets; ESR—erythrocyte sedimentation rate; CRP—C-reactive protein; Na$^+$—sodium; K$^+$—potassium; NT-proBNP—N-terminal prohormone of brain natriuretic peptide; TSH—thyrotropin; Peak VO$_2$—peak oxygen consumption; VE/VCO$_2$ slope—minute ventilation/carbon dioxide production; PETCO$_2$—partial pressure of end-tidal carbon dioxide; LVEF—left ventricle ejection fraction; ACE-I—angiotensin-converting enzyme inhibitors; ARB—angiotensin II receptor blocker; ARNI—angiotensin receptor neprilysin inhibitor; MRA—mineralocorticoid receptor antagonist.

sST2 concentration was measured in all patients. The mean value of sST2 was 45.5 ± 40.8 ng/mL. The SST2 level was significantly lower in the group of the survivors compared to that of the group of non-survivors (38.8 ± 32.0 ng/mL vs. 60.5 ± 53.3 ng/mL; *p* = 0.0029). During median follow up (2.7 years), 34 (30.9%) patients died and 63 (57.3%) patients achieved composite endpoint (all-cause death, hospitalization or intravenous diuretics requirement, or heart transplantation). During the follow-up period, 50 patients (45.5%) required hospitalization or intravenous diuretics. SST2 levels were significantly lower in the group of survivors as compared to the group of non-survivors (38.8 ± 32.0 ng/mL vs. 60.5 ± 53.3 ng/mL; *p* = 0.0029) (Figure 1). Based on collected data, the ROC curve was calculated for all-cause death, and the reference cut-off point for sST2 was determined to be 45.818 pg/mL (AUC 0.676, *p* = 0.0009) (Figure 2). According to the cut-off point, the study group was divided into two groups according to the sST2 values.

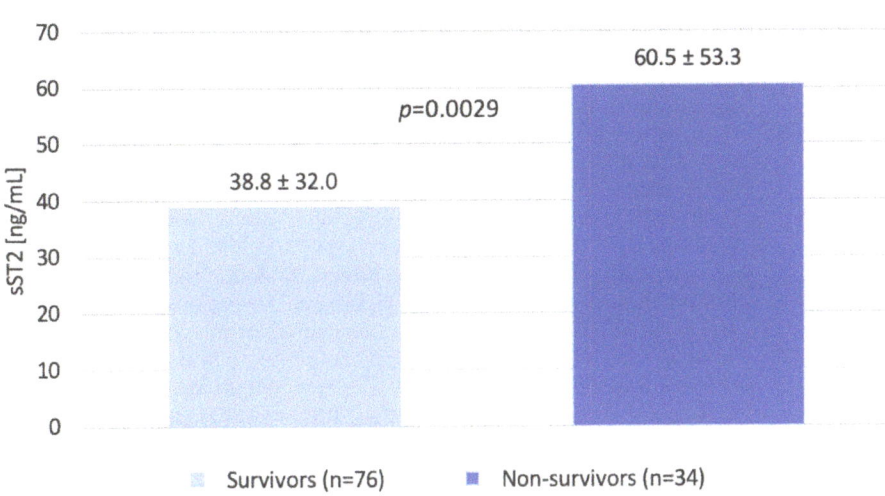

Figure 1. The mean values of sST2.

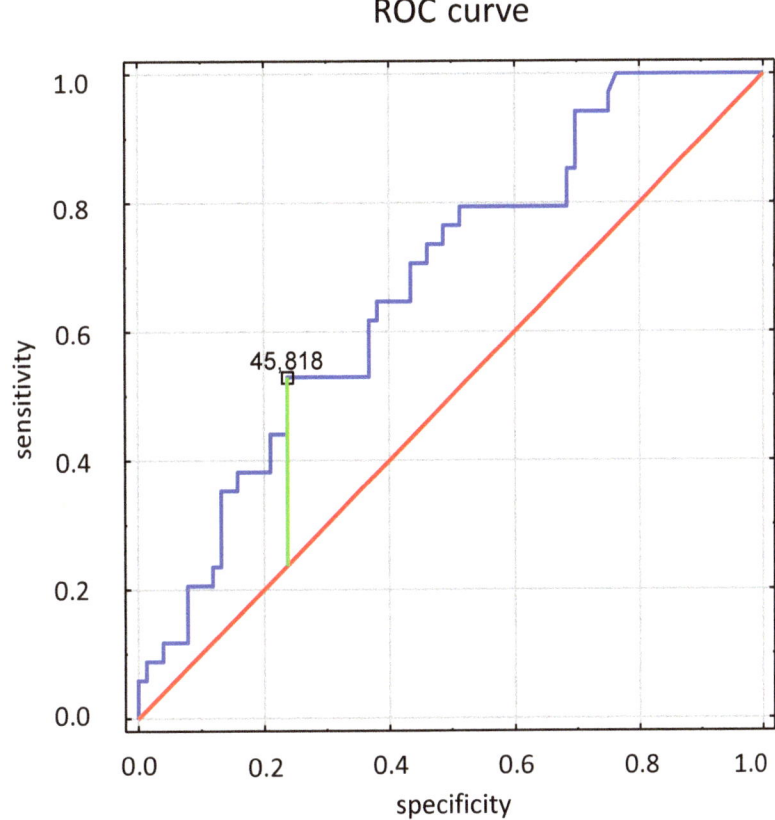

Figure 2. The reference cut-off point for sST2 for all-cause death.

There were significant differences in the inflammatory parameters between groups. Patients with an sST2 concentration >45.8 pg/mL had significantly higher WBC (8.3 ± 2.0 vs. 7.3 ± 1.9; p = 0.0020), neutrophils (5.6 ± 1.5 vs. 4.6 ± 1.5, p = 0.0005), monocytes (0.6 ± 0.3 vs. 0.5 ± 0.1, p = 0.0016), and CRP values (8.2 ± 12.4 vs. 2.6 ± 3.1, p < 0.001) compared to those of the people with a lower concentrations. In addition, in this group the sodium concentration was significantly lower (137.9 ± 3.2 vs. 140.0 ± 2.1; p = 0.0005). The study groups differed in liver function parameters. AST and GGTP levels were significantly higher in patients with higher concentration of sST2. Significantly higher levels of BNP and NT-proBNP were observed in patients with higher levels of sST2. For BNP, the levels were 740.8 ± 779.5 pg/mL vs. 286.7 ± 318.9 pg/mL (p < 0.001), respectively, and for NT-proBNP, the levels were 3862.9 ± 5909.3 pg/mL vs. 1477.0 ± 1702.8 pg/mL (p < 0.001), respectively.

The LVEFs were similar in both groups (Table 2). In data obtained from cardiopulmonary exercise testing, we noticed significantly lower peak VO$_2$ values (1.3 ± 0.3 L/min vs. 1.6 ± 0.6 L/min; p = 0.0030) in the subgroup of patients with higher sST2 protein values in comparison with those of the subgroup of people with sST2 ≤ 45.8 pg/mL. There were also significant differences in the VE/VCO$_2$ slope, which was higher in patients with higher sST2 levels (35.7 ± 8.1 vs. 31.6 ± 6.9; p = 0.0188), and PETCO$_2$, which was lower in patients with higher sST2 levels.

Table 2. Comparison of clinical and biochemical parameters between groups according to sST2 value.

Parameter	sST2 ≤ 45.8 (n = 74)	sST2 > 45.8 (n = 36)	p
Age (years)	53.0 ± 11.7	53.4 ± 11.0	0.7488
Men	89.20%	91.70%	0.6844
BMI (kg/m^2)	28.9 ± 4.8	26.6 ± 3.7	**0.0146**
SBP (mmHg)	110.1 ± 16.3	104.9 ± 12.6	0.1808
DBP (mmHg)	72.2 ± 9.5	66.9 ± 8.1	**0.0090**
LVEF (%)	23.9 ± 8.0	21.9 ± 7.6	0.2595
Duration of HF (months)	101.5 ± 92.1	83.7 ± 72.7	0.5155
Etiology of HF—CAD	49%	56%	0.2950
Etiology of HF—DCM	50%	39%	0.2950
NYHA class	2.4 ± 0.6	2.6 ± 0.5	0.2164
ICD	50%	39%	0.2950
CRT-D	50%	39%	0.2950
Comorbidities			
AF	9.50%	30.60%	**0.0039**
Arterial hypertension	47.30%	38.90%	0.405
Diabetes mellitus type II	21.60%	33.30%	0.3411
Thyroid disease	17.60%	22.20%	0.56
COPD	12.20%	13.90%	0.7987
Smoking at admission	10.80%	16.70%	0.5877
Smoking history	54.10%	55.60%	0.5877

Table 2. Cont.

Parameter	sST2 ≤ 45.8 (n = 74)	sST2 > 45.8 (n = 36)	p
Biochemical parameters			
WBC (10^9/L)	7.3 ± 1.9	8.3 ± 2.0	**0.002**
RBC (10^{12}/L)	4.7 ± 0.4	4.8 ± 0.6	0.9368
HGB (mmol/L)	9.0 ± 0.7	8.9 ± 0.8	0.2094
RDW (%)	15.0 ± 4.9	15.8 ± 1.7	**0.0001**
PLT (10^9/L)	197.8 ± 51.2	210.3 ± 55.7	0.2437
ESR (mm/h)	8.2 ± 7.3	12.4 ± 14.4	0.422
CRP (mg/L)	2.6 ± 3.1	8.2 ± 12.4	**<0.001**
Na^+ (mmol/L)	140.0 ± 2.1	137.9 ± 3.2	**0.0005**
K^+ (mmol/L)	4.6 ± 2.4	4.2 ± 0.6	0.1958
Creatinine (umol/L)	101.2 ± 25.0	106.7 ± 21.9	0.2872
Fasting glucose (mmol/L)	6.5 ± 2.7	6.4 ± 1.7	0.5155
NT-proBNP (pg/mL)	1477.0 ± 1702.8	3862.9 ± 5909.3	**<0.001**
TSH (uIU/mL)	1.9 ± 1.7	2.0 ± 1.8	0.9671
CPET parameters			
Peak VO_2 (mL/kg/min)	18.1 ± 5.5	15.8 ± 4.1	0.062
Peak VO_2 (L/min)	1.6 ± 0.6	1.3 ± 0.3	**0.003**
Peak VO_2 (%)	56.5 ± 16.0	49.5 ± 15.2	**0.0095**
VE/VCO_2 slope	31.6 ± 6.9	35.7 ± 8.1	**0.0188**
$PETCO_2$ (mmHg)	34.6 ± 5.8	29.7 ± 6.0	**<0.001**
Medications			
Beta-blocker	98.70%	97.20%	0.5993
ACE-I/ARB	82.40%	83.30%	0.9066
ARNI	12.20%	5.60%	0.2784
MRA	86.50%	88.90%	0.7227
Loop diuretic	89.20%	91.70%	0.6844

BMI—body mass index; SBP—systolic blood pressure; DBP—diastolic blood pressure; NYHA—New York Heart Association; HF—heart failure; CAD—coronary artery disease; DCM—dilated cardiomyopathy; ICD—implantable cardioverter-defibrillator; CRT-D—cardiac resynchronization therapy defibrillator; AF—atrial fibrillation; COPD—chronic obstructive pulmonary disease; WBC—white blood cells; RBC—red blood cells; HGB—hemoglobin; RDW—red blood cell distribution width; PLT—platelets; ESR—erythrocyte sedimentation rate; CRP—C-reactive protein; Na^+—sodium; K^+—potassium; NT-proBNP—N-terminal prohormone of brain natriuretic peptide; TSH—thyrotropin; Peak VO_2—peak oxygen consumption; VE/VCO_2 slope—minute ventilation/carbon dioxide production; $PETCO_2$—partial pressure of end-tidal carbon dioxide; LVEF—left ventricle ejection fraction; ACE-I—angiotensin-converting enzyme inhibitors; ARB—angiotensin II receptor blocker; ARNI—angiotensin receptor neprilysin inhibitor; MRA—mineralocorticoid receptor antagonist.

The probability of the primary endpoint depending on sST2 concentration was estimated using Kaplan–Meier curves (Figure 3). The Kaplan–Meier plot graphically shows that the probability of survival was significantly higher in the group of patients with low sST2 concentrations as compared to that of the group with high sST2 values ($p = 0.0027$).

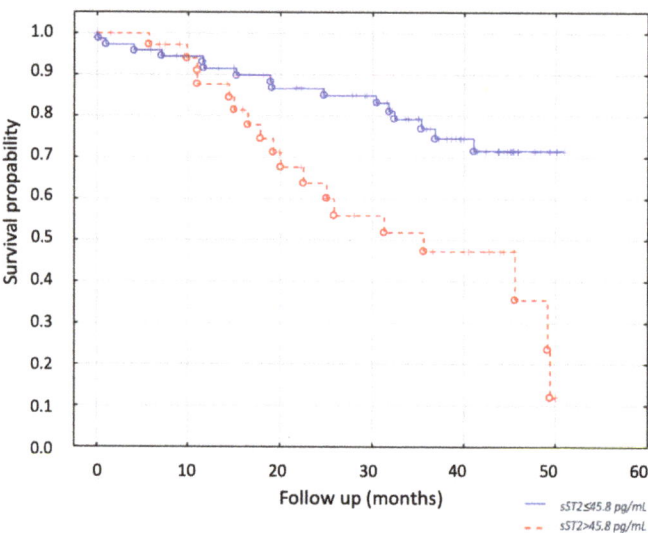

Figure 3. Influence of sST2 concentration on survival.

In order to assess the influence of covariates on the relationship between sST2 concentration and the occurrence of the endpoint, multivariate analysis was performed. Based on the obtained and predicted relationships between dependent and independent variables, the following parameters were tested using multivariate models: systolic blood pressure, sST2, RDW, CRP, NT-proBNP, albumin, etiology of HF, peak oxygen uptake VE/VCO$_2$ slope, and PETCO$_2$.

Based on a multivariate regression model, it was shown that the independent predictors of death in stable patients with HFrEF were: peak oxygen uptake expressed in ml/kg/min (hazard ratio, 0.89; p = 0.0308), red blood cell distribution width (RDW) (hazard ratio, 1.10; p = 0.0074), and the concentration of sST2 (hazard ratio, 1.00; p = 0.0206).

4. Discussion

The most important finding of the presented analysis is that an increased concentration of sST2 is an independent risk factor for all-cause death in a group of patients with stable HFrEF.

Cardiovascular diseases, including HF, are the leading cause of morbidity and mortality in the industrialized world [14]. Despite significant progress in the understanding of pathophysiology, the introduction of prophylaxis, and modern therapeutic methods, HF is still a significant health and social problem which leads to a deterioration in the quality of life of patients and increased mortality. New markers are constantly being researched to help in the diagnosis and monitoring of patients with HF, as well as to help in identifying the group with the highest risk level. sST2 protein is gaining attention as a potential tool for monitoring the treatment of CHF and as a prognostic marker in this group due to its involvement in inflammatory processes and mechanical overload, as well as remodeling and fibrosis [12]. It was noted that sST2 concentrations in CHF patients were generally higher than they were in the healthy population [15].

In recent years, there has been an increased interest in this biomarker. Initially, sST2 was used in the assessment of HF decompensation, and also recently, for patients with CHF.

In the course of the PRIDE study (Pro-Brain Natriuretic Peptide Investigation of Dyspnea in the Emergency Department) [15], sST2 levels were measured in almost six hundred patients who were admitted to the emergency department due to dyspnea with suspected HF. It should be emphasized that the study group included both people with and without HF. The study [15] showed a significantly higher concentration of sST2 in the group of patients with dyspnea due to HF and the relationship between the concentration of sST2 and mortality in both groups of patients (higher concentrations of the biomarker suggest a higher risk of death). The publication by Mueller et al. [16] presents similar results: increased sST2 concentrations at the initial presentation in patients with acute heart failure (AHF) indicate an increased risk of death in the future; however, no cut-off value was reported for prognostic significance.

The presented study showed that the concentration of sST2 is an independent predictor of all-cause death in the group of patients with stable HFrEF. In patients who died during the observation, a significantly higher concentration of sST2 protein was found at the point of enrollment in the study (60.5 ± 53.3 pg/mL vs. 38.8 ± 32.0 pg/mL; $p = 0.0029$). Higher baseline sST2 levels are a strong predictor of death; 50% of patients with sST2 > 45.8 pg/mL died, while 21.6% patients from the group with lower levels died ($p = 0.0025$). Our study is one of the few studies that assessed the prognostic value of sST2 in patients with HFrEF, and the endpoint was assessed as death due to all causes.

Additionally, in a meta-analysis [17] conducted on a group of over 4000 patients, it was shown that the concentration of sST2 is an independent predictor of death from general and cardiovascular causes and an independent risk factor for HF-related hospitalization. Several fundamental differences between the Emdin study [17] and the one presented here should be emphasized. The study group [17] consisted of patients with HFrEF and heart failure with preserved ejection fraction (HFpEF) and with a higher mean age than that in our own study (68 years vs. 53 years). The follow-up was comparable in length to that in our own study (average 2.4 years), but the cut-off value for the sST2 level as a risk factor for death from all causes, death from cardiovascular causes, or hospitalization due to HF was 28 ng/mL. This is lower than it is in the analysis performed here, but the endpoints were different. It should be noted that research on sST2 is ongoing, and no specific cut-off value has been established for it as a prognostic indicator. Soluble ST2, together with galectin 3, is a parameter indicated by American experts as a promising marker that is helpful for predicting hospitalization and death in patients with HF, which may have even greater prognostic value than natriuretic peptides do. However, the 2017 update of the American College of Cardiology/American Heart Association HF guidelines [18] did not specify a cut-off value for sST2 for predicting the occurrence of death or adverse cardiovascular events. It seems that the purpose of including sST2 and galectin 3 in the guidelines [18,19] was to highlight the potential utility of these markers and to encourage further research in this area.

The long-term follow-up performed by Emdin et al. [17] assessed three endpoints of death from all causes, death from cardiovascular causes, and hospitalization due to HF. Cardiovascular deaths were not analyzed in our study as these data were not available. During the entire follow-up (mean 2.45 years) in this analysis, 34 patients (30.9%) died. This mortality rate is comparable to those in the analysis [17], where the all-cause mortality was 31% and the cardiovascular mortality was 22%. In the analyzed study, the inclusion criterion was a stable clinical condition at least 4 weeks before inclusion in the study. Despite the relatively good initial clinical condition of patients (mean NYHA 2.4), the applied optimal treatment, and the vast majority (82%) of patients having implanted cardioverter-defibrillators, mortality was not low. Another observation shows that the prognosis of patients is still not good, despite the use of an appropriate treatment. It seems that in patients with HF who are in a stable clinical condition, stabilization is only apparent.

Patients with higher sST2 concentrations had a higher percentage of diagnosed atrial fibrillation ($p = 0.0039$). The pathophysiologically increased hemodynamic load causes atrial distension, which is a well-known cause of the development of AF. The same mechanism can also stimulate sST2 secretion. A study by Chen et al. [20] showed that people with AF have a significantly higher concentration of soluble ST2 proteins than people with a sinus rhythm do. Higher sST2 concentrations in patients with AF are probably due to higher atrial pressures and higher heart rates than those in patients with a sinus rhythm [20].

Surprisingly, despite significantly higher concentrations of natriuretic peptides in non-surviving patients than the concentrations of those who survived, natriuretic peptides were not found to be an independent risk factor for all-cause mortality. They are recognized risk factors used in the diagnosis of HF [1] and prognosis of these patients [21–24]. Although significant correlations were observed between the concentrations of natriuretic peptides and the concentrations of sST2, people with higher sST2 concentrations have higher BNP ($p < 0.001$) and NT-proBNP ($p = 0.001$) values.

In patients with higher concentrations of sST2, we found higher levels of inflammatory markers. The available literature has shown that high concentrations of CRP protein and other markers have significant prognostic and therapeutic implications in HF [25]. In a study by Dupuy et al. [26] assessing sST2 and CRP levels in patients with CHF ($n = 178$), a combined multi-marker model including sST2 and CRP was presented. This study showed that the combination of high CRP (>6.4 mg/L) and elevated sST2 (>47.6 ng/mL) dramatically increased the risk of mortality, and a further association with NT-proBNP provided no additional information [26]. The cut-off point for sST2 in the study [26] was similar to the values determined in this analysis. The publication [26] confirmed that high sST2 values in combination with an elevated CRP are associated with an increased risk of all-cause or cardiovascular mortality, which is consistent with the results of this analysis.

Another parameter that is a well-established marker of poor prognosis for patients with HF is hyponatremia (defined as serum sodium concentration <135 mEq/L) [27–30]. In the study analyzed here, significant differences in sodium concentrations between the groups were observed. Significantly lower sodium concentrations were measured in subjects with higher sST2 values (137.9 ± 3.2 vs. 140.0 ± 2.1; $p = 0.0005$). The results obtained in the current analysis are consistent with those in available publications, which have proven that low sodium concentrations are associated with a higher mortality rate and are a predictor of hospitalization of patients with HF. No analyses on the correlation between sodium and sST2 concentrations were found in the available literature.

Our study had some limitations. According to ESC 2021 guidelines, sodium-glucose co-transporter 2 (SGLT2) inhibitors added to a therapy with ACE-I/ARNI/beta-blocker/MRA reduced the risk of CV death and worsening HF in patients with HFrEF. Our patients were involved in the study before these guidelines were published. Second, we analyzed a small number of patients in a single-center study. The majority of our study group were men; therefore, the cut-off point for sST2 in the group of women with HFrEF should be interpreted with caution.

5. Conclusions

sST2 protein concentration is an independent risk factor for all-cause death in patients with stable HF with reduced left ventricular ejection fraction. We suppose that sST2 may help to distinguish the group of patients with HFrEF who are at the highest risk, which will allow the better optimization of treatment and intensification of medical care in the form of more frequent check-ups of these patients.

Author Contributions: Conceptualization, M.D. and M.K.-O.; data curation, M.D., M.L. and E.S.-M.; formal analysis, M.D., M.K.-O., M.L. and E.S.-M.; funding acquisition, M.D., M.K.-O. and E.S.-M.; investigation, M.D., F.S. and H.K.; methodology, M.D., M.K.-O., J.M. and F.S.; project administration, M.D.; resources, M.D. and M.K.-O.; software, J.M. and F.S.; supervision, M.D. and E.S.-M.; validation, M.D., M.K.-O., M.L. and E.S.-M.; visualization, M.D., M.K.-O., J.M., F.S., H.K. and M.L.; writing—original draft, M.D., M.K.-O., J.M., F.S. and H.K.; writing—review and editing, M.D., M.K.-O., M.L. and E.S.-M. All authors have read and agreed to the published version of the manuscript.

Funding: This research received no external funding.

Institutional Review Board Statement: The study was conducted in accordance with the Declaration of Helsinki, and approved by the Institutional Review Board (or Ethics Committee) of Poznan University of Medical Sciences (No. 378/19).

Informed Consent Statement: Informed consent was obtained from all subjects involved in the study.

Data Availability Statement: The data presented in this study are available on request from the corresponding author.

Conflicts of Interest: The authors declare no conflict of interest.

References

1. McDonagh, T.A.; Metra, M.; Adamo, M.; Gardner, R.S.; Baumbach, A.; Böhm, M.; Burri, H.; Butler, J.; Čelutkienė, J.; Chioncel, O.; et al. 2021 ESC Guidelines for the diagnosis and treatment of acute and chronic heart failure. *Eur. Heart J.* **2021**, *42*, 3599–3726. [CrossRef]
2. Mosterd, A.; Hoes, A.W. Clinical epidemiology of heart failure. *Heart* **2007**, *93*, 1137–1146. [CrossRef]
3. Ambrosy, A.P.; Fonarow, G.C.; Butler, J.; Chioncel, O.; Greene, S.J.; Vaduganathan, M.; Nodari, S.; Lam, C.S.P.; Sato, N.; Shah, A.N.; et al. The global health and economic burden of hospitalizations for heart failure: Lessons learned from hospitalized heart failure registries. *J. Am. Coll. Cardiol.* **2014**, *63*, 1123–1133. [CrossRef]
4. Bui, A.L.; Horwich, T.B.; Fonarow, G.C. Epidemiology and risk profile of heart failure. *Nat. Rev. Cardiol.* **2011**, *8*, 30–41. [CrossRef]
5. Miller, K.D.; Siegel, R.L.; Lin, C.C.; Mariotto, A.B.; Kramer, J.L.; Rowland, J.H.; Stein, K.D.; Alteri, R.; Jemal, A. Cancer treatment and sur-vivorship statistics, 2016. *CA Cancer J. Clin.* **2016**, *66*, 271–289. [CrossRef]
6. Giamouzis, G.; Kalogeropoulos, A.; Georgiopoulou, V.; Laskar, S.; Smith, A.L.; Dunbar, S.; Triposkiadis, F.; Butler, J. Hospitalization Epidemic in Patients with Heart Failure: Risk Factors, Risk Prediction, Knowledge Gaps, and Future Directions. *J. Card. Fail.* **2011**, *17*, 54–75. [CrossRef]
7. Schmitz, J.; Owyang, A.; Oldham, E.; Song, Y.; Murphy, E.; McClanahan, T.K.; Zurawski, G.; Moshrefi, M.; Qin, J.; Li, X.; et al. IL-33, an Interleukin-1-like Cytokine that Signals via the IL-1 Receptor-Related Protein ST2 and Induces T Helper Type 2-Associated Cytokines. *Immunity* **2005**, *23*, 479–490. [CrossRef]
8. Coglianese, E.E.; Larson, M.G.; Vasan, R.S.; Ho, J.E.; Ghorbani, A.; McCabe, E.L.; Cheng, S.; Fradley, M.G.; Kretschman, D.; Gao, W.; et al. Distribution and Clinical Correlates of the Interleukin Receptor Family Member Soluble ST2 in the Framingham Heart Study. *Clin. Chem.* **2012**, *58*, 1673–1681. [CrossRef]
9. Zhu, J.; Ruan, Z.; Zhu, L. Correlation between Serum LP-PLA2 and sST2 Levels and the Condition of Patients with Acute Heart Failure and Their Prognostic Value. *Evid.-Based Complement. Altern. Med.* **2021**, *2021*, 8267776. [CrossRef]
10. Sun, Y.; Feng, L.; Hu, B.; Dong, J.; Zhang, L.; Huang, X.; Yuan, Y. Prognostic Value of β1 Adrenergic Receptor Autoantibody and Soluble Suppression of Tumorigenicity-2 in Patients with Acutely Decompensated Heart Failure. *Front. Cardiovasc. Med.* **2022**, *9*, 75. [CrossRef]
11. Ponikowski, P.; Voors, A.A.; Anker, S.D.; Bueno, H.; Cleland, J.G.F.; Coats, A.J.S.; Falk, V.; González-Juanatey, J.R.; Harjola, V.P.; Jankowska, E.A.; et al. 2016 ESC Guidelines for the diagnosis and treatment of acute and chronic heart failure of the European Society of Cardiology (ESC)Developed with the special contribution of the Heart Failure Association (HFA) of the ESC. *Eur. Heart J.* **2016**, *37*, 2129–2200.
12. Dieplinger, B.; Januzzi, J.L.; Steinmair, M.; Gabriel, C.; Poelz, W.; Haltmayer, M.; Mueller, T. Analytical and clinical evaluation of a novel high-sensitivity assay for measurement of soluble ST2 in human plasma—The Presage™ ST2 assay. *Clin. Chim. Acta* **2009**, *409*, 33–40. [CrossRef]
13. Lang, R.M.; Badano, L.P.; Mor-Avi, V.; Afilalo, J.; Armstrong, A.; Ernande, L.; Flachskampf, F.A.; Foster, E.; Goldstein, S.A.; Kuznetsova, T.; et al. Recommendations for cardiac chamber quantification by echocardiography in adults: An update from the American So-ciety of Echocardiography and the European Association of Cardiovascular Imaging. *J. Am. Soc. Echocardiogr.* **2015**, *28*, 233–271. [CrossRef]
14. Virani, S.S.; Alonso, A.; Benjamin, E.J.; Bittencourt, M.S.; Callaway, C.W.; Carson, A.P.; Chamberlain, A.M.; Chang, A.R.; Cheng, S.; Delling, F.N.; et al. Heart Disease and Stroke Statistics-2020 Update: A Report from the American Heart Association. *Circulation* **2020**, *141*, e139–e596. [CrossRef]
15. Januzzi, J.L.; Peacock, W.F.; Maisel, A.S.; Chae, C.U.; Jesse, R.L.; Baggish, A.L.; O'Donoghue, M.; Sakhuja, R.; Chen, A.A.; van Kimmenade, R.R.; et al. Measurement of the Interleukin Family Member ST2 in Patients with Acute Dyspnea: Results From the PRIDE (Pro-Brain Natriuretic Peptide Investigation of Dyspnea in the Emergency Department) Study. *J. Am. Coll. Cardiol.* **2007**, *50*, 607–613. [CrossRef]
16. Mueller, C.; Laule-Kilian, K.; Christ, A.; Rocca, H.P.B.; Perruchoud, A.P. Inflammation and long-term mortality in acute congestive heart failure. *Am. Heart J.* **2006**, *151*, 845–850. [CrossRef]
17. Emdin, M.; Aimo, A.; Vergaro, G.; Bayes-Genis, A.; Lupón, J.; Latini, R.; Meessen, J.; Anand, I.S.; Cohn, J.N.; Gravning, J.; et al. sST2 Predicts Outcome in Chronic Heart Failure Beyond NT-proBNP and High-Sensitivity Troponin T. *J. Am. Coll. Cardiol.* **2018**, *72*, 2309–2320. [CrossRef]
18. Yancy, C.W.; Jessup, M.; Bozkurt, B.; Butler, J.; Casey, D.E., Jr.; Colvin, M.M.; Drazner, M.H.; Filippatos, G.S.; Fonarow, G.C.; Givertz, M.M.; et al. 2017 ACC/AHA/HFSA Focused Update of the 2013 ACCF/AHA Guideline for the Management of Heart

Failure: A Report of the American College of Cardiology/American Heart Association Task Force on Clinical Practice Guidelines and the Heart Failure Society of America. *J. Am. Coll. Cardiol.* **2017**, *70*, 776–803.
19. Heidenreich, P.A.; Bozkurt, B.; Aguilar, D.; Allen, L.A.; Byun, J.J.; Colvin, M.M.; Deswal, A.; Drazner, M.H.; Dunlay, S.M.; Evers, L.R.; et al. 2022 AHA/ACC/HFSA Guideline for the Management of Heart Failure: A Report of the American College of Cardiolo-gy/American Heart Association Joint Committee on Clinical Practice Guidelines. *Circulation* **2022**, *145*, e895–e1032. [CrossRef]
20. Chen, C.; Qu, X.; Gao, Z.; Zheng, G.; Wang, Y.; Chen, X.; Li, H.; Huang, W.; Zhou, H. Soluble ST2 in Patients with Nonvalvular Atrial Fibrillation and Prediction of Heart Failure. *Int. Heart J.* **2018**, *59*, 58–63. [CrossRef]
21. Harjola, V.-P.; Mullens, W.; Banaszewski, M.; Bauersachs, J.; Brunner-La Rocca, H.P.; Chioncel, O.; Collins, S.P.; Doehner, W.; Filippatos, G.S.; Flammer, A.J.; et al. Organ dysfunction, injury and failure in acute heart failure: From pathophysiology to diagnosis and management. A review on behalf of the Acute Heart Failure Committee of the Heart Failure Association (HFA) of the European Society of Cardiology (ESC). *Eur. J. Heart Fail.* **2017**, *19*, 821–836. [CrossRef]
22. Oremus, M.; Don-Wauchope, A.; McKelvie, R.; Santaguida, P.L.; Hill, S.; Balion, C.; Booth, R.; Brown, J.A.; Ali, U.; Bustamam, A.; et al. BNP and NT-proBNP as prognostic markers in persons with chronic stable heart failure. *Heart Fail Rev.* **2014**, *19*, 471–505. [CrossRef]
23. Maeda, K.; Tsutamoto, T.; Wada, A.; Mabuchi, N.; Hayashi, M.; Tsutsui, T.; Ohnishi, M.; Sawaki, M.; Fujii, M.; Matsumoto, T.; et al. High levels of plasma brain natriuretic peptide and interleukin-6 after optimized treatment for heart failure are independent risk factors for morbidity and mortality in patients with congestive heart failure. *J. Am. Coll. Cardiol.* **2000**, *36*, 1587–1593. [CrossRef]
24. Maisel, A.S.; Duran, J.M.; Wettersten, N. Natriuretic Peptides in Heart Failure: Atrial and B-type Natriuretic Peptides. *Heart Fail Clin.* **2018**, *14*, 13–25. [CrossRef]
25. Cesari, M.; Penninx, B.W.; Newman, A.B.; Kritchevsky, S.B.; Nicklas, B.J.; Sutton-Tyrrell, K.; Rubin, S.M.; Ding, J.; Simonsick, E.M.; Harris, T.B.; et al. Inflammatory markers and onset of cardiovascular events: Results from the Health ABC study. *Circulation* **2003**, *108*, 2317–2322. [CrossRef]
26. Dupuy, A.M.; Curinier, C.; Kuster, N.; Huet, F.; Leclercq, F.; Davy, J.M.; Cristol, J.P.; Roubille, F. Multi-Marker Strategy in Heart Failure: Combination of ST2 and CRP Predicts Poor Outcome. *PLoS ONE* **2016**, *11*, e0157159. [CrossRef]
27. Keddis, M.T.; El-Zoghby, Z.; Kaplan, B.; Meeusen, J.W.; Donato, L.J.; Cosio, F.G.; Steidley, D.E. Soluble ST2 does not change cardiovascular risk prediction compared to cardiac troponin T in kidney transplant candidates. *PLoS ONE* **2017**, *12*, e0181123. [CrossRef]
28. Bavishi, C.; Ather, S.; Bambhroliya, A.; Jneid, H.; Virani, S.S.; Bozkurt, B.; Deswal, A. Prognostic Significance of Hyponatremia Among Ambulatory Patients with Heart Failure and Preserved and Reduced Ejection Fractions. *Am. J. Cardiol.* **2014**, *113*, 1834–1838. [CrossRef]
29. Bettari, L.; Fiuzat, M.; Shaw, L.K.; Wojdyla, D.M.; Metra, M.; Felker, G.M.; O'connor, C.M. Hyponatremia and Long-Term Outcomes in Chronic Heart Failure—An Observational Study from the Duke Databank for Cardiovascular Diseases. *J. Card. Fail.* **2012**, *18*, 74–81. [CrossRef]
30. Gheorghiade, M.; Abraham, W.T.; Albert, N.M.; Stough, W.G.; Greenberg, B.H.; O'Connor, C.M.; She, L.; Yancy, C.W.; Young, J.; Fonarow, G.C.; et al. Relationship between admission serum sodium concentration and clinical outcomes in patients hospitalized for heart failure: An analysis from the OPTIMIZE-HF registry. *Eur. Heart J.* **2007**, *28*, 980–988. [CrossRef]

Disclaimer/Publisher's Note: The statements, opinions and data contained in all publications are solely those of the individual author(s) and contributor(s) and not of MDPI and/or the editor(s). MDPI and/or the editor(s) disclaim responsibility for any injury to people or property resulting from any ideas, methods, instructions or products referred to in the content.

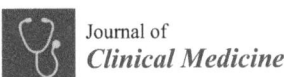

Article

Prognostic Value of Plasma Catestatin Concentration in Patients with Heart Failure with Reduced Ejection Fraction in Two-Year Follow-Up

Łukasz Wołowiec [1,*], Joanna Banach [1], Jacek Budzyński [2], Anna Wołowiec [3], Mariusz Kozakiewicz [3], Maciej Bieliński [4], Albert Jaśniak [1], Agata Olejarczyk [2] and Grzegorz Grześk [1]

[1] Department of Cardiology and Clinical Pharmacology, Faculty of Health Sciences, Collegium Medicum in Bydgoszcz, Nicolaus Copernicus University, 87-100 Toruń, Poland; albertjasniak@gmail.com (A.J.); ggrzesk@cm.umk.pl (G.G.)

[2] Department of Vascular and Internal Diseases, Faculty of Health Sciences, Collegium Medicum in Bydgoszcz, Nicolaus Copernicus University, 87-100 Toruń, Poland; jb112233@cm.umk.pl (J.B.); agatuh@gmail.com (A.O.)

[3] Department of Geriatrics, Division of Biochemistry and Biogerontology, Faculty of Health Sciences, Collegium Medicum in Bydgoszcz, Nicolaus Copernicus University, 87-100 Toruń, Poland; anna.wolowiec@cm.umk.pl (A.W.); markoz@cm.umk.pl (M.K.)

[4] Department of Clinical Neuropsychology, Faculty of Health Sciences, Collegium Medicum in Bydgoszcz, Nicolaus Copernicus University, 85-094 Bydgoszcz, Poland; maciejb@cm.umk.pl

* Correspondence: lukaswolowiec111@gmail.com

Abstract: The primary objective of the study was to evaluate the prognostic value of measuring plasma catestatin (CST) concentration in patients with heart failure with reduced ejection fraction (HFrEF) as a predictor of unplanned hospitalization and all-cause death independently and as a composite endpoint at 2-year follow-up. The study group includes 122 hospitalized Caucasian patients in NYHA classes II to IV. Patients who died during the 24-month follow-up period ($n = 44$; 36%) were significantly older on the day of enrollment, were more likely to be in a higher NYHA class, had lower TAPSE, hemoglobin concentration, hematocrit, and platelet count, higher concentrations of CST, NT-proBNP, troponin T, creatinine, and glucose, and higher red cell distribution width value and leukocyte and neutrocyte count than patients who survived the follow-up period. Plasma catestatin concentration increased with NYHA class ($R = 0.58$; $p < 0.001$) and correlated significantly with blood NT-proBNP concentration ($R = 0.44$; $p < 0.001$). We showed that higher plasma catestatin concentration increased the risk of all-cause death by more than five times. Plasma CST concentration is a valuable prognostic parameter in predicting death from all causes and unplanned hospitalization in patients with HFrEF.

Keywords: catestatin; heart failure; HFrEF; biomarker; biomarkers for heart failure prognosis

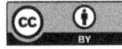

1. Introduction

The prevalence of heart failure (HF) in the general adult population is 1–3% [1] and increases rapidly after the age of 75, reaching 20% in people aged 70–80 [1]. These statistics seem to be constantly increasing, which can be associated with the phenomenon of aging populations and improved survival after acute myocardial infarction. HF is the most common cause of hospitalization in patients >65 years of age [2]. The high rate of expensive readmissions is one of the main causes of the economic burden of HF, which is a major challenge for health care systems worldwide.

The annual health care cost per HF patient in Germany in 2011 was EUR 3150 per year and increases with the severity of the disease according to the New York Heart Association (NYHA) classification of heart failure. Compared to the EUR 2474 spent per patient in NYHA class I, the cost in NYHA class II increases by 14%, in NYHA class III by 48%, and in NYHA class IV by 71% [3]. The cost of hospitalization ranges from 74 to 90% of the total direct and indirect expenditure related to HF [1,3]. In 2012, the American Heart Association estimated a 2.5-fold increase in the medical costs of HF in the United States, from USD 20.9 billion in 2012 to USD 53.1 billion in 2030, and an approximately 2-fold increase in HF cases in men [4]. These statistics show the great importance of precise risk stratification enabling early identification of subgroups of patients with the worst prognosis in order to quickly implement optimal treatment methods. Due to the important role of markers in HF [5–11] and the need to discover new ones, we decided to evaluate the clinical usefulness of measuring plasma catestatin (CST) in patients with HFrEF as a predictor of unplanned hospitalization and all-cause death independently and as a composite endpoint at a two-year follow-up.

CST is a bioactive peptide composed of 21 amino acids that is formed as a result of the cleavage of the prohormone chromogranin A (CgA). CgA occurs in the chromaffin cells of the adrenal medulla and in other cells of the neuroendocrine and nervous systems, from where it is secreted from secretory granules by autocrine signaling, or together with catecholamines (CA) by exocytosis. CgA has also been detected in endomyocardial biopsy material in people with heart disease [12], as well as in normal heart tissues where a decrease in CST concentration was observed with age [13]. Unlike CA, which is rapidly degraded in plasma, CST is highly stable and is considered a useful marker of sympathetic activation. Previous clinical studies show that the level of CST can remain elevated for some time despite treatment and alleviation of HF symptoms [14].

In 1997, Mahata et al. synthesized 15 peptides that make up CgA and showed that only one of them inhibited nicotine-induced CA secretion [15]. They named the discovered peptide CST because of its high ability to inhibit CA release [16] by binding to nicotinic acetylcholine receptors that block Na+ uptake [15]. A direct antagonistic effect of CST on β-adrenergic receptors with a hypotensive effect has also been described [17]. In humans, plasma CST concentrations have been shown to increase in situations of marked sympathetic stimulation, such as in critically ill patients [18]. High plasma CST concentrations have been found in people with HF [5] due to coronary artery disease [19], hypertension [20], dilated cardiomyopathy [12], hypertrophic cardiomyopathy [12], and valvular disease [12]. Plasma CgA concentrations have been shown to increase with the advancement of various human heart diseases [21].

The main cardioprotective properties of CST can be derived from the in vivo vasodilatation observed. The beneficial afterload reduction resulting from vasodilatation appears to be a multifactorial mechanism mediated by histamine, along with a reduction in reactive oxygen species availability and stimulation of nitric oxide production [22]. CST activates the β2-ARs-PI3K-eNOs-NO (β2-adrenergic receptors-phosphoinositide 3-kinases-endothelial nitric oxide synthase-nitric oxide) signaling pathway in endocardial endothelial cells, which play a role in myocardial remodeling. In connection with the above, it can be assumed that the inhibition of the fibrosis process by CST occurs through increased production of NO [23,24]. Another anti-hypertrophic mechanism for modulating coronary vascular tone is blocked by the CST receptor for endothelin-1 [25,26]. Additional mechanisms may include pleiotropism-limiting metabolic syndromes, including research-proven anti-inflammatory, anti-atherosclerotic, anti-diabetic and anti-apoptotic effects. CST suppresses TNF-α-elicited expression of inflammatory cytokines and adhesion molecules by activating angiotensin-converting enzyme 2 (ACE2), [27], induces glucose uptake and Glut4 (Glucose transporter type 4) translocation in cardiomyocytes [28], upregulates insulin-induced Akt phosphorylation, reduces endoplasmic reticulum stress (ERS) and increases insulin sensitivity [29]. CST inhibits ERS-induced cardiomyocyte apoptosis by simultaneously activating the β2-adrenergic receptor and the PKB/Akt (phosphatidylinositol 3-kinase/protein kinase B) pathway [30]. CST supports the immunosuppression of macrophages and differentiates their phenotypes towards anti-inflammatory behavior [31], promotes the oxidation of fatty acids and their flow from adipose tissue to the liver, and lowers plasma leptin levels by resensitizing receptors to leptin [32].

The main aim of our study was to assess the usefulness of determining plasma CST concentration, collected within 24 h of admission to the hospital or first contact with a health professional at a clinic, as a predictor of unplanned hospitalization and all-cause mortality independently and as a CE in the group of patients with HFrEF at a two-year follow-up.

2. Materials and Methods

2.1. Study Population

The study group consisted of 122 Caucasian patients with HFrEF in NYHA classes II-IV, who were either treated on an outpatient basis or hospitalized in the Department of Cardiology and Clinical Pharmacology or the Department of Vascular and Internal Diseases at the Nicolaus Copernicus University Collegium Medicum University Hospital No. 2 in Bydgoszcz, Poland, for planned medical procedures, some of whom were on the elective list of patients waiting for heart transplantation. Outpatient patients were under the care of the Cardiology Clinic and Heart Failure Clinic operating in the department. The diagnosis of HFrEF was based on the criteria of the European Society of Cardiology (ESC). Patients received optimal pharmacological treatment for each patient in accordance with the ESC guidelines [33].

The study protocol was approved by the Bioethical Committee of the Nicolaus Copernicus University in Toruń at the Collegium Medicum in Bydgoszcz. Each patient signed an informed consent form after obtaining detailed information about the purpose and scope of the study. The criteria for inclusion in the study were age over 18, heart failure diagnosed according to the criteria included in the guidelines of the European Society of Cardiology, heart failure class II-IV according to NYHA, left ventricular ejection fraction (LVEF) $\leq 40\%$ assessed during the current hospitalization or up to 6 months earlier. The exclusion criteria were sepsis or shock from any cause on admission to hospital, acute coronary syndrome, recent (<3 months) myocardial infarction or stroke, active neoplasm, autoimmune diseases, impaired liver function (INR without oral anticoagulation > 1.5, bilirubin total > 1.5 mg%, or 3 times the upper limit of normal for ALT), corticosteroid therapy, decompensated diabetes mellitus requiring treatment with intravenous insulin infusion, chronic inflammatory bowel diseases, or recent (<3 months) surgery.

2.2. Catestatin Determination

All biochemical analytes were routinely collected upon admission to the Department of Cardiology and Clinical Pharmacology and Clinical Pharmacology or the Department of Vascular and Internal Diseases. Blood specimens were collected by venipuncture into 5 mL tubes containing tripotassium EDTA. Plasma blood was centrifuged ($3000\times g$ for 15 min) and aliquoted into Eppendorf tubes. Samples were stored at a temperature of $-80\ ^\circ$C until biochemical analysis was performed. The plasma catestatin concentration was measured by an enzyme immunoassay (ELISA) commercial kit, Human Catestatin EIA, from RayBiotech, (Norcross, GA, USA), catalog number EIA-CAT-1, dilution factor $12 \times$ for human, reproducibility intra-assay: CV and < 10%, and inter-assay: CV and < 15%. According to the manufacturer, the reactivity with human CST is 100%. The analytical sensitivity of the method (lower detection limit for the test) is 0.5 ng/mL. The results were obtained with a SPECTROstar Nano (BMG LABTECH) spectrophotometric reader using MARS data analysis software version 2.41. The marker was evaluated at the 450 nm wavelength. The results were read from the calibration curve prepared for the analyzer used in the study. All analyses were performed in accordance with the manufacturer's instructions.

2.3. Statistical Analysis

Statistical analysis was conducted using the licensed version of the statistical analysis software STATISTICA version 13.1 (TIBCO Software, Inc., Palo Alto, CA, USA, 2017). The statistical significance level was set at a *p*-value of < 0.05. The normal distribution of the study variables was analyzed using the Kolmogorov–Smirnov test. The results were presented as the mean ± standard deviation; median, interquartile range (IQR); or as a frequency (*n*, %) of the categorical variables. The statistical significance of differences between groups was verified using the Student's *t*-test, the Mann–Whitney U-test, and one-factorial ANOVA with Bonferroni post hoc test for quantitative variables (when more than one comparison was necessary) and the Chi-square test for qualitative variables. We also used a ROC curve with the lowest Youden index and the AUC to determine the cut-off values of the parameters measured. Kaplan–Meir analysis and Cox hazards regression model were performed to determine the factors affecting the risk of all-cause mortality and all-cause readmission. Spearman's correlation was also used. The logistic regression method was applied to determine the risk of measured outcome occurrence associated with respective cut-offs of the parameters studied.

3. Results

3.1. Clinical Characteriscits

Of 122 consecutive HFrEF patients, 78 were admitted to the hospital with exacerbation (including de novo heart failure) and 44 were in stable condition. Although there is no precise definition of heart failure exacerbation, we decided to include only patients who demonstrated certain dynamics of increasing hypervolaemia, and ultimately urged these patients to seek medical care. Low-output states were excluded from the study, as in our opinion in initial stages it is difficult to make a clear distinction between plain HF exacerbation with hypotension and developing cardiogenic shock, a classic form of acute heart failure. Two patients were not included in the final analysis due to lack of survival data after 12 months of follow-up. Patients who died during the follow-up period ($n = 44$, 36%) were significantly older at the day of enrollment, were more likely to be in a higher NYHA class, and had lower TAPSE, hemoglobin concentration, hematocrit, and platelets count, higher concentrations of catestatin, NT-proBNP, troponin T, creatinine, and glucose, and higher RDW values and leukocyte and neutrocyte counts than patients who survived the follow-up period (Table 1). Pharmacotherapy differed between groups, mainly in relation to ASA (acetylsalicylic acid), NOACs (non-vitamin K oral anticoagulants), and diuretic use (Table 2).

Table 1. Comparison of baseline parameters studied in patients who died or survived during long-term follow-up.

Parameter (Unit)	Death ($n = 44$)	Survived ($n = 76$)	*p*
Male sex	34 (77.27)	59 (77.63)	0.964
Age (years)	69.91 ± 13.74	55.53 ± 12.80	<0.001
NYHA (II. III. IV)	2 (4.55) 17 (38.64) 25 (56.82)	37 (48.68) 26 (34.21) 13 (17.11)	<0.001
Readmission (%)	27 (61.36)	26 (34.21)	0.004
TAPSE (mm)	16.89 ± 3.90	19.64 ± 4.80	<0.001
EF (%)	24.82 ± 8.63	27.88 ± 8.28	0.057
Etiology (DCM/ICM)	20 (45.45) 24 (54.55)	50 (65.79) 26 (34.21)	0.030
BMI (kg/m^2)	28.39 ± 5.93	29.87 ± 5.99	0.194
DM	19 (43.18)	30 (39.47)	0.693
HT	26 (59.09)	37 (48.68)	0.275
AF	27 (61.36)	32 (42.11)	0.390
ICD/CRT-d	26 (58.09)	62 (61.58)	0.005

Table 1. Cont.

Parameter (Unit)	Death (n = 44)	Survived (n = 76)	p
NT-proBNP (pg/mL)	9620.80 ± 8883.64	3703.30 ± 6165.45	<0.001
Catestatin (ng/mL)	38.94 ± 33.30	24.53 ± 15.66	0.002
TNT (µg/L)	0.06 ± 0.07	0.03 ± 0.05	0.003
Creatinine (mg/dL)	1.40 ± 0.46	1.09 ± 0.32	<0.001
hsCRP (mg/L)	16.91 ± 27.43	11.55 ± 30.01	0.333
HB (g/dL)	12.45 ± 2.40	14.07 ± 1.66	<0.001
HCT (%)	37.94 ± 7.18	41.63 ± 4.26	<0.001
PLT (1000/mm^3)	182.39 ± 72.27	211.20 ± 68.02	0.031
RDW (%)	16.65 ± 2.86	14.38 ± 1.87	<0.001
WBC (1000/mm^3)	8.71 ± 2.91	7.74 ± 2.25	0.043
NEUT (1000/mm^3)	7.21 ± 5.22	4.84 ± 1.81	<0.001

TAPSE: tricuspid annular plane systolic excursion; EF: ejection fraction; DCM/ICM: dilated cardiomyopathy/ischemic cardiomyopathy; BMI: body mass index; DM: diabetes mellitus; HT: hypertension, AF: atrial fibrillation; ICD/CRT-d: implantable cardioverter-defibrillator/cardiac resynchronization therapy with defibrillator; NT-proBNP: N-terminal fragment of B-type natriuretic propeptide; TNT: troponin t; hsCRP: high-sensitivity CRP; HB: hemoglobin; HCT: hematocrit; PLT: platelets; RDW: red cell distribution width; WBC: white blood cells; NEUT: neutrophils.

Table 2. Differences regarding received pharmacotherapy among patients who died or survived throughout long-term follow-up.

Parameter (Unit)	Death (n = 44)	Survived (n = 76)	p
ACEI	22 (50.00)	51 (67.11)	0.065
ARB	8 (18.18)	17 (22.37)	0.590
ASA	5 (11.36)	28 (36.84)	0.002
BB	39 (88.64)	70 (92.11)	0.530
Digoxin	5 (11.36)	8 (10.53)	0.888
Statin	35 (79.55)	58 (76.32)	0.686
Ivabradine	4 (9.09)	7 (9.21)	0.983
VKA	9 (20.45)	19 (25.00)	0.574
Amiodarone	8 (18.18)	6 (7.89)	0.092
NOAC	23 (52.27)	16 (21.05)	<0.001
Spironolactone	14 (31.82)	31 (40.79)	0.332
Eplerenone	13 (29.55)	35 (46.07)	0.076
Furosemide	8 (18.18)	22 (28.95)	0.192
Torasemide	29 (65.91)	28 (36.84)	0.002
HCTZ	2 (4.55)	8 (10.53)	0.257

ACEI: angiotensin-converting-enzyme inhibitors; ARB: angiotensin II receptor blockers; ASA: acetylsalicylic acid; VKA: vitamin K antagonist; NOAC: non-vitamin K antagonist oral anticoagulants; HCTZ: hydrochlorothiazide.

Plasma catestatin concentration increased with NYHA class (R = 0.58; $p < 0.001$); however, those relationships were weaker than those obtained for NT-proBNP (R = 0.66; $p < 0.001$). Plasma catestatin concentration correlated significantly with blood NT-proBNP concentration (R = 0.44; $p < 0.001$) and did not reach significance for BMI.

3.2. Plasma Catestatin Concentration as a Factor for Discriminating among HFrEF Patients

In the next step of analysis, using ROC curve analysis, we determined how catestatin cut-off predicted risk of all-cause mortality during long-term follow up. Compared to patients with lower plasma catestatin concentrations, those with plasma catestatin concentrations higher than or equal to the established cut-off (27.94 pmol/L; AUC, 95% CI: 0.706, 0.609–0.803, $p < 0.001$) were significantly older and had higher prevalence of advanced NYHA class, all-cause readmission, mortality, and composite endpoints, and shorter survival time (Table 2). Statistically significant differences between groups mentioned also included: prevalence of hypertension, history of CIED implantation, TAPSE, NT-proBNP, troponin T, creatinine, glucose, neutrocyte percentage, hemoglobin, and hematocrit (Table 3). Correlations between catestatin and selected parameters are presented in Table 4.

Table 3. Parameters studied in HFrEF patients in relation to plasma catestatin concentration.

Parameter (Unit)	Catestatin ≥ 27.94 (n = 47)	Catestatin < 27.94 (n = 73)	p
Male sex	34 (72.34%)	59 (80.82)	0.342
Age (years)	69.71 ± 14.42	55.08 ± 11.94	<0.001
NYHA (II. III. IV)	1 (2.13%) 22 (46.81%) 24 (51.06%)	38 (52.05) 21 (28.77) 14 (19.18)	<0.001
Readmission (%)	26 (55.32%)	27 (36.99)	0.048
All-causes death	26 (55.32%)	16 (21.92)	<0.001
Composite endpoint	39 (82.98%)	31 (42.47)	<0.001
Survival time (days)	587.53 ± 371.82	710.37 ± 202.32	0.02
TAPSE (mm)	16.51 ± 3.57	20.04 ± 4.01	<0.001
EF (%)	27.10 ± 9.25	26.82 ± 8.10	0.860
Etiology (DCM/ICM)	23 (48.94%) 24 (51.10%)	47 (64.38) 26 (35.62)	0.057
BMI (kg/m^2)	29.51 ± 5.36	29.22 ± 6.33	0.789
DM	24 (51.06%)	25 (34.25)	0.066
HT	30 (68.83%)	33 (45.21)	0.029
AF	28 (59.57%)	30 (41.10)	0.003
ICD/CRTD	20 (42.55%)	66 (90.41)	<0.001
NT-proBNP (pg/mL)	9423.00 ± 7950.45	3405.51 ± 6609.79	<0.001
TNT (µg/L)	0.07 ± 0.08	0.02 ± 0.03	<0.001
Creatine (mg/dL)	1.41 ± 0.46	1.06 ± 0.30	<0.001
Glucose (mg/dL)	141.29 ± 46.15	120.01 ± 41.00	<0.01
hsCRP (mg/L)	17.40 ± 26.13	10.82 ± 30.44	0.219
HB (g/dL)	12.31 ± 2.17	14.19 ± 1.75	<0.001
HCT (%)	37.45 ± 5.85	42.03 ± 5.03	<0.001
PLT (1000/mm^3)	197.73 ± 77.99	203.59 ± 65.44	0.655
RDW (%)	16.23 ± 2.59	14.57 ± 2.24	<0.001
WBC (1000/mm^3)	8.56 ± 2.51	7.78 ± 2.54	0.096
NEUT (%)	70.90 ± 10.93	62.47 ± 11.81	<0.001
NEUT (1000/mm^3)	6.03 ± 2.53	5.45 ± 4.19	0.389
ACEI	19 (40.43%)	54 (73.97)	<0.001

Table 3. Cont.

Parameter (Unit)	Catestatin ≥ 27.94 (n = 47)	Catestatin < 27.94 (n = 73)	p
ARB	10 (21.27%)	15 (20.55)	0.804
ASA	10 (21.27%)	23 (31.51)	0.179
BB	38 (80.85%)	71 (97.26)	<0.01
Digoxin	4 (8.51%)	9 (12.33)	0.469
Statin	35 (74.47%)	58 (79.54)	0.611
Ivabradine	3 (6.38%)	8 (10.96)	0.365
VKA	7 (14.89%)	21 (14.29)	0.063
NOAC	24 (51.06%)	15 (53.06)	<0.001
Amiodarone	8 (17.02%)	6 (8.22)	0.171
Spironolactone	18 (38.30%)	27 (36.99)	0.843
Eplerenone	6 (12.77%)	42 (57.53)	<0.001
Furosemide	10 (21.27%)	20 (27.40)	0.542
Torsemide	28 (59.57%)	29 (39.73)	0.034
HCTZ	1 (2.13%)	9 (12.33)	0.043

NYHA: New York Heart Association Functional Classification; TAPSE: tricuspid annular plane systolic excursion; EF: ejection fraction; DCM: dilated cardiomyopathy; ICM: ischemic cardiomyopathy; BMI: body mass index; DM: diabetes mellitus; HT: hypertension AF: atrial fibrillation; ICD/CRTD: implantable cardioverter-defibrillator cardiac resynchronization therapy with defibrillator; NT-proBNP: N-terminal fragment of prohormone B-type natriuretic propeptide; TNT: troponin t; hsCRP: high-sensitivity CRP; HB: hemoglobin; HCT: hematocrit; PLT: platelets; RDW: red cell distribution width; WBC: white blood cells; NEUT: neutrophils; ACEI: angiotensin-converting-enzyme inhibitors; ARB: angiotensin II receptor blockers; ASA: acetylsalicylic acid; BB: beta adrenergic receptor antagonists; VKA: vitamin K antagonist; NOAC: non-vitamin K antagonist oral anticoagulants; HCTZ: hydrochlorothiazide.

Table 4. Correlations between catestatin and selected parameters, n = 120.

Parameter (Unit)	Correlations between Catestatin and Selected Parameters	
	r	p
Age (years)	0.3711	<0.001
EF (%)	−0.0663	0.472
BMI (kg/m^2)	−0.0004	0.997
TAPSE (mm)	−0.2793	0.002
NT-proBNP (pg/mL)	0.4390	<0.001
TNT (µg/L)	0.2195	0.016
Creatinine (mg/dL)	0.2937	0.001
hsCRP (mg/L)	0.1120	0.223
Glucose (mg/dL)	0.1970	0.031
HB (g/dL)	−0.2483	0.006

EF: ejection fraction; BMI: body mass index; TAPSE: tricuspid annular plane systolic excursion; NT-proBNP: N-terminal fragment of prohormone B-type natriuretic propeptide; TNT: troponin t; hsCRP: high-sensitivity CRP; HB: hemoglobin.

3.3. Survival Analysis

Using cut-offs values obtained for catestatin ROC analysis for prediction of all-cause mortality, readmission, and composite endpoint occurrence, we performed Kaplan–Meier analysis, which confirmed the influence of catestatin on long-term prognosis among HFrEF patients. We found that higher plasma catestatin concentration increased the risk of all-cause death by more than five-times (Figures 1–3).

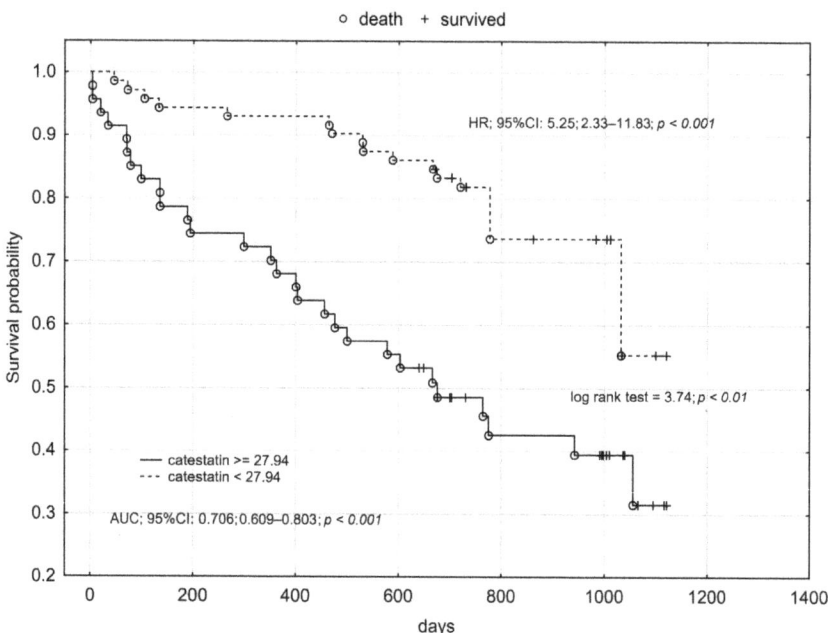

Figure 1. Kaplan–Meier analysis for all-cause mortality of HFrEF patients in relation to plasma catestatin concentration.

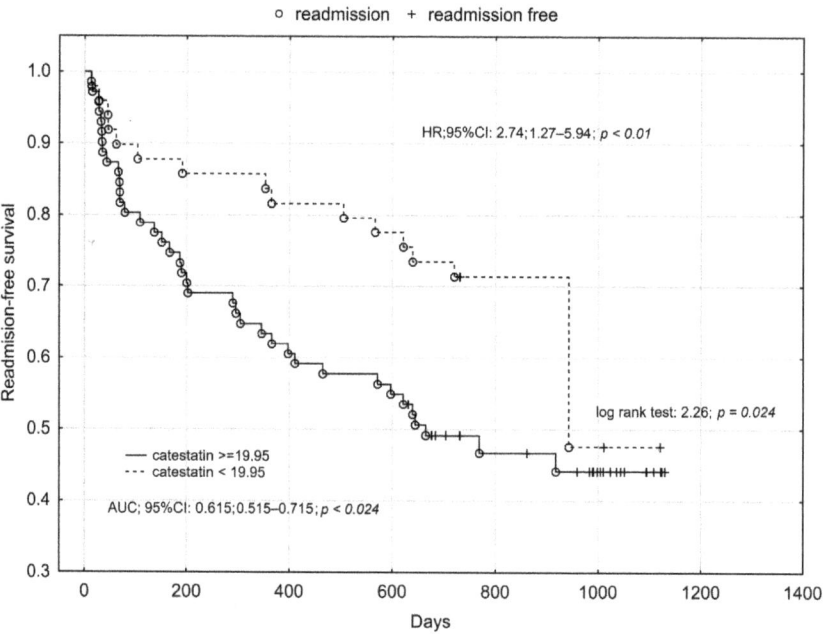

Figure 2. Kaplan–Meier analysis for all-cause readmission of HFrEF patients in relation to plasma catestatin concentration.

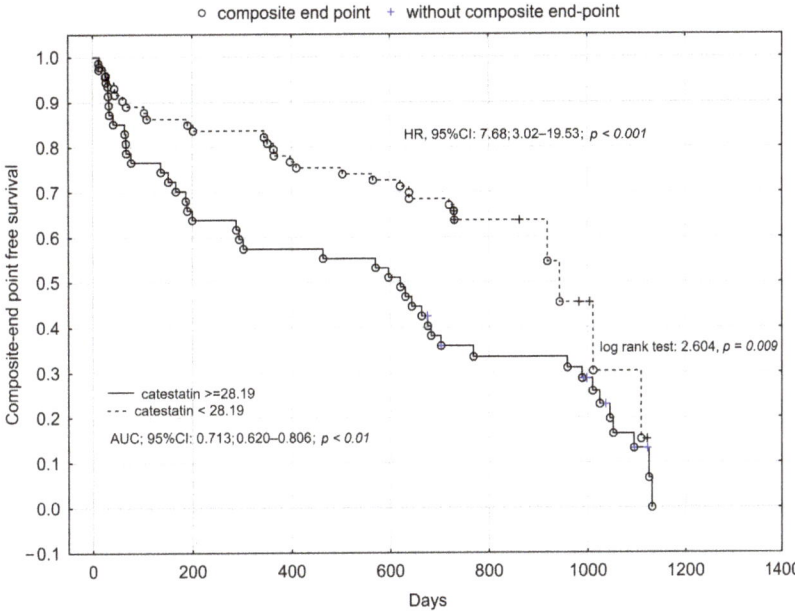

Figure 3. Kaplan–Meier analysis for composite endpoint of HFrEF patients in relation to plasma catestatin concentration.

Using the Cox regression proportional hazard method, we tried to determine independent risk factors for measured outcomes among HFrEF patients. We achieved statistically significant regression models; however, none of the biomarkers included in the model reached statistical significance (Tables 5–7, Figure 4).

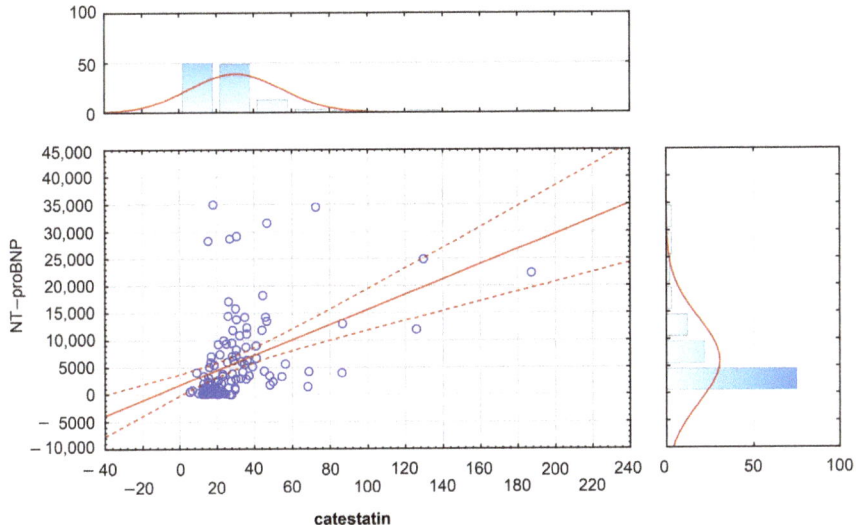

Figure 4. Correlation of catestatin and NT-proBNP, R = 0.439, $p < 0.001$. Individual data points represent Box-Cox transformed values. Solid red line—regression line estimated from the sample population. Red dashed lines—confidence curves = 0.95.

Table 5. Cox proportional hazard regression model for death prediction, chi^2 = 48.69; $p < 0.001$.

Parameter (Unit)	HR	p
NT-proBNP (pg/mL)	1.00; 1.00–1.00	0.437
Catestatin (ng/mL)	1.004; 0.994–1.014	0.414
Creatinine (mg/dL)	1.791; 0.942–3.406	0.076
Age (years)	1.054; 1.025–1.085	<0.001
BMI (kg/m^2)	0.924; 0.864–0.988	0.021
LVEF (%)	0.950; 0.912–0.990	0.014

NT-proBNP: N-terminal fragment of prohormone B-type natriuretic propeptide; BMI: body mass index; LVEF: left ventricle ejection fraction.

Table 6. Cox proportional hazard regression model for prediction of all-cause readmission, chi^2 = 26.51; $p < 0.001$.

Parameter (Unit)	HR. 95%CI	p
NT-proBNP (pg/mL)	1.00; 1.00–1.00	0.047
Catestatin (ng/mL)	1.003; 0.99–1.02	0.664
Creatinine (mg/dL)	1.58; 0.85–2.94	0.153
Age (years)	1.03; 1.01–1.05	0.018
BMI (kg/m^2)	0.97; 0.92–1.03	0.315
LVEF (%)	0.96; 0.93–0.99	0.047

NT-proBNP: N-terminal fragment of prohormone B-type natriuretic propeptide; BMI: body mass index; LVEF: left ventricle ejection fraction.

Table 7. Cox proportional hazard regression model for prediction of composite endpoint, chi^2 = 48.29; $p < 0.001$.

Parameter (Unit)	HR. 95%CI	p
NT-proBNP (pg/mL)	1.00; 0.99–1.00	0.151
Catestatin (ng/mL)	1.01; 0.99–1.01	0.316
Creatinine (mg/dL)	1.48; 0.85–2.56	0.163
Age (years)	1.04; 1.02–1.06	<0.001
BMI (kg/m^2)	0.95; 0.91–1.00	0.063
LVEF (%)	0.95; 0.92–0.98	0.004

NT-proBNP: N-terminal fragment of prohormone B-type natriuretic propeptide; BMI: body mass index; LVEF: left ventricle ejection fraction.

Annotation: X: catestatin; $n = 120$, mean = 29.813250; standard deviation = 24.573521; max = 187.230000; min = 5.520000; Y: NT-BNP; $n = 120$; mean = 5873.05000; standard deviation = 7789.3915; max = 35,000.00000; min = 24.000000; NT-BNP= 1724.8 + 139.14* catestatin; correlation: R = 0.43896; confidence interval = 0.95.

4. Discussion

Although all our patients were carefully qualified as having a reduced left ventricular ejection fraction, the presence of patients in various clinical conditions presenting both stable and exacerbated HFrEF courses reduced the homogeneity of the study group. Another limitation was their single ethnicity and the performance of the study in one research center, which reduced the representativeness of the tested marker for the world population. It should also be noted that the methodology used did not allow determining whether plasma CST concentration provided additional prognostic information compared to natriuretic peptides (NP), or whether adding CST to other known prognostic factors improved the prognostic model. However, the concentration of CST increased significantly with the NYHA class (R = 0.58; $p < 0.001$) and correlated significantly with the currently used markers of heart failure, including TNT (R = 0.22; $p = 0.016$) and NT-proBNP (R = 0.44; $p < 0.001$), but did not show a significant correlation with BMI (R = -0.0004; $p = 0.997$). According to information published in the 2021 ESC Guidelines for the diagnosis and treatment of acute and chronic heart failure [33,34], NP levels may be disproportionately low in obese individuals. Moreover, the cited guidelines emphasize that there are many causes of elevated NP levels, both cardiovascular and non-cardiovascular, that may reduce their diagnostic accuracy. Some examples of these are ischemic stroke, renal failure, cirrhosis, COPD, and anemia. Due to the differences in the correlation with BMI between CST and pro-BNP, the potential prognostic advantage of CST over NP should be the subject of future analyses in the obese population with the above diseases. CST is also not a specific marker for HFrEF, and other clinical situations with increased sympathetic activation in particular critical conditions including sepsis [18] may alter the prognostic value in the context of HF. Despite these limitations, our results indicate that elevated CST levels were associated with a worse prognosis among patients with HfrEF in the long-term follow-up. CST allows a statistically significant regression model, and the clinical usefulness of plasma CST concentration as a prognostic factor in HfrEF patients was not worse than NT-proBNP. Although CST did not reach statistical significance with regard to rehospitalizations, we found that a higher plasma CST concentration increased the risk of all-cause death by more than five times. The obtained data allowed identifying stable patients with the worst prognosis. Patients with high CST levels may benefit from systematic follow-up and may be candidates for more aggressive treatment. Changes in CST concentrations are the result of a number of related pathomechanisms involved in HF, such as oxidative stress, chronic inflammation, excessive activation of the immune system and sympathetic nervous system (SNS), and their consequences. Issues related to the pleiotropic effect of CST demonstrate that after the action of the factor leading to the change in the force of myocardial contraction, there must be a number of compensatory mechanisms that are interconnected and interdependent, and the circulatory system decompensates when a specific critical point is reached. CST is therefore part of a complex neurohumoral feedback system and is secreted as a counterregulatory peptide that attenuates excess catecholamines and SNS activity. Higher levels of this peptide in plasma may indirectly reflect increased neurohumoral load and dysfunctional baroreceptor control.

Since the incorporation of natriuretic peptide assessment into routine clinical practice, many reliable markers of heart failure have been tested with varying results. Considering the high residual risk, reflecting the multifaceted pathophysiology of heart failure, even with their significant clinical role, natriuretic peptides seem to be insufficient. Thus, a multi-marker approach may help to refine therapeutic strategies and allow treatment to be tailored to the individual clinical and biochemical profile of each patient with HF.

The analysis of the collected data suggests that higher plasma CST values in patients with HFrEF were associated with a worse prognosis in the long-term follow-up. Although the risks for CE, all-cause mortality, and all-cause rehospitalization depend on a constellation of various factors, CST provides a statistically significant regression model, which is why we consider CST to be a useful marker that is competitive with currently used markers of heart failure.

Our 2020 publication examining the CST level in the population of Polish patients with HFrEF showed that the difference in plasma CST concentration between healthy individuals and properly treated patients with stable CHF may be minimal or nonexistent [5].

Since CST reflects SNS mobilizations, in accordance with our assumptions, adding patients with an exacerbated clinical course of HFrEF and de novo HFrEF to the study group resulted in an increase in the CST level in correlation with the severity of NH symptoms according to the NYHA classification and a decrease in the LVEF value. This is because, like NT-proBNP, CST turns out to be a marker of hemodynamic instability. Available literature data on the usefulness of this marker during follow-up and the effect of pharmacotherapy on catestatin concentrations are minimal. A review of the current literature reveals four clinical studies examining plasma catestatin levels [5,14,35,36] and one examining serum [37] catestatin levels in various stages of HF.

Despite the use of a smaller and less homogeneous study group in terms of LVEF, conclusions similar to our findings were reached by Borovac et al. [37] in a non-randomized cross-sectional clinical trial conducted from January 2018 to February 2019. The study included 95 individuals with signs and symptoms of NYHA class II–IV HF. All patients were in a clinical exacerbation described as acute decompensated heart failure (ADHF), most with HFrEF ($n = 39$, 43.4%) and others with HFpEF (heart failure with preserved ejection fraction) ($n = 31$, 34.4%) or HFmrEF (heart failure with mid-range ejection fraction) ($n = 20$ 22.2%). Contrary to other studies, Borovac et al. determined serum CST levels. In their multivariable linear regression analysis, CST independently correlated with NYHA class ($\beta = 0.491$, $p < 0.001$), waist-to-hip ratio (WHR) ($\beta = -0.237$, $p = 0.026$), HbA1c ($\beta = -0.235$, $p = 0.027$), LDL ($\beta = -0.231$, $p = 0.029$), non-HDL cholesterol ($\beta = -0.237$, $p = 0.026$), hs-cTnI ($\beta = -0.221$, $p = 0.030$), heart rate on admission, and resting heart rate ($\beta = -0.201$, $p = 0.036$ and $\beta = -0.242$, $p = 0.030$) and was associated with most echocardiographic parameters, but did not differ between patients with reduced, mild, or preserved LVEF (7.74 ± 5.64 vs. 5.75 ± 4.19 vs. 5.35 ± 2.77 ng/mL, $p = 0.143$, respectively). ROC analysis showed that the plasma level of CST was comparable in terms of diagnostic efficacy and provided significantly higher AUC values in patients who died than in patients who survived compared to traditional biomarkers such as NT-proBNP and hs-cTnI [37]. Due to the compensatory effect of CST on adverse neurohumoral activation, which is especially pronounced in ischemic diseases, the researchers obtained significantly higher CST concentrations in patients with ADHF associated with myocardial infarction (MI) compared to patients without MI. Although the CST levels observed by Borovac et al. were not significantly different between the three LVEF phenotypes, the investigators noted a clear trend towards higher CST levels in HFrEF patients, although statistical significance was not reached, most likely due to limited sample size. In addition, circulating CST levels were highest in the NYHA IV subgroup, followed by NYHA III, and lowest in the NYHA II subgroup. This study is in line with our results. Other researchers (Liu et al.) [14] who included patients of all NYHA classes in their studies obtained similar concentrations in class I and II and significantly higher concentrations in class III and IV.

Only one of the available studies (Zhu et al.) [35], despite collecting the largest study group ($n = 300$), obtained a surprising (because inconsistent with other studies) inverse relationship between CST and clinical advancement of HF. The authors assessed CST levels in different phases of HF and the diagnostic utility of CST as a potential biomarker for the detection of asymptomatic HF in stage B according to the American Heart Association (AHA). In the group of 300 patients (stage B: $n = 76$, age 68.58 ± 8.63, LVEF $54.95 \pm 9.82\%$), it was shown that the concentration of CST decreased from stage A, through B, to C. The cut-off point for the CST stage B HF detection value was 19.73 ng/mL, with a sensitivity of 90% (higher than BNP in this study) and a specificity of 50.9%. Contrary to our results, Zhu et al. found no correlation between CST and BNP concentration ($R = 0.107$, $p = 0.150$ versus $R = 0.61$, $p < 0.001$). According to the authors, asymptomatic patients with stage B HF will benefit most from regular follow-up and therapeutic intervention; as observed in this group, a decrease in catestatin levels may precede full-blown HF.

Comparing the group from our study with Zhu et al.'s stage C (the most appropriate comparison in terms of the occurrence of symptoms and the largest representation in the study group), significant differences should be emphasized regarding the optimal pharmacological treatment (beta-blocker 90.83% vs. 86.2%, ACEi or sartan 81.6% vs. 72.4%, spironolactone or eplerenone 77.5% vs. no data). After increasing the size of the study group, which in the current study also includes patients with exacerbation of HF and with de novo HF, we obtained divergent conclusions to Zhu et al. and a positive correlation of CST with clinical severity of HF.

Although our study did not assess the effect of treatment on HF marker levels, interesting observations come from Liu et al. [14]. In their research, plasma CST concentrations did not decrease significantly despite treatment and alleviation of HF symptoms, while plasma BNP concentrations decreased significantly. This finding may suggest retention of residual catecholaminergic activity, which is not reflected in the reduction of circulating natriuretic peptides. Optimal pharmacological treatment should include further suppression of the sympathetic component until normalization of CST levels. The difference in concentration between markers may also result from distinct mechanisms underlying the production, distribution and excretion of both markers. Simultaneous measurement of different markers may provide broader insight into different aspects of HFrEF pathophysiology and increase the prognostic value of the tests performed, which should be the basis of modern risk stratification.

Even if our analysis of patients with an exacerbation included clinically stable individuals, which reduced the homogeneity of the study group, the results obtained allowed us to isolate stable patients with the worst prognosis, which allowed for the early application of more aggressive treatment methods.

Future studies should focus on measuring CST among similar cohorts of HF patients, taking into account their clinical parameters, variability of CgA metabolism, medical history and pharmacotherapy (including new-generation drugs such as levosimendan [38] and proprotein convertase subtilisin/kexin 9 inhibitors [39]). Such actions will make it possible to estimate the range of norms of the persistent sympathetic component in patients with HF, assess the effectiveness of treatment and direct further pharmacotherapy to the residual neurohormonal disease.

The limitations of the present study were the relatively small study population and the lack of assessment of possible changes in chromogranin A proteolysis disorders in the study group.

5. Conclusions

The prognostic model for the study endpoints—unplanned hospitalization, all-cause death, and the composite endpoint—depends on a constellation of different factors. Higher plasma catestatin concentration was associated with worse prognosis in HFrEF patients during long-term follow-up and increased the risk of all-cause death by more than five times. Plasma CST concentration increased significantly with NYHA class ($R = 0.58$; $p < 0.001$) and correlated significantly with currently used HF markers, including TNT ($R = 0.22$; $p = 0.016$) and NT-proBNP ($R = 0.44$; $p < 0.001$). Patients with high CST levels may benefit from systematic follow-up and may be candidates for more aggressive treatment. Due to the differences in the correlation with BMI between CST and NT-proBNP and the disproportionately low levels of natriuretic peptides in the obese population, future studies should evaluate the possible prognostic advantage of CST in overweight cardiac patients.

Author Contributions: Ł.W.: Conceptualization, Formal analysis, Methodology, Writing—Original Draft, Project administration Supervision; J.B. (Joanna Banach): Writing—Original Draft Project administration Data Curation; J.B. (Jacek Budzyński): Formal analysis Writing—Original Draft, Visualization; A.W.: Writing—Original Draft Resources Data Curation; M.K.: Writing—Original Draft Resources Data Curation; M.B.: Writing—Original Draft Resources Data Curation; A.J.: Writing—Original Draft, Visualization; A.O.: Writing—Original Draft Resources Data Curation; G.G.: Conceptualization, Methodology, Writing—Original Draft, Supervision. All authors have read and agreed to the published version of the manuscript.

Funding: This research received no external funding.

Institutional Review Board Statement: Study protocol was in compliance with the principles of the Declaration of Helsinki. The study protocol was approved by the Bioethical Committee of the Nicolaus Copernicus University in Toruń at the Collegium Medicum in Bydgoszcz, Poland (KB 591/2016).

Informed Consent Statement: Informed consent was obtained from all subjects involved in the study.

Data Availability Statement: All data used to support the finding of this study are available from the corresponding author upon request.

Conflicts of Interest: The authors declare no conflict of interest.

References

1. Savarese, G.; Becher, P.M.; Lund, L.H.; Seferovic, P.; Rosano, G.M.C.; Coats, A.J.S. Global burden of heart failure: A comprehensive and updated review of epidemiology. *Cardiovasc. Res.* **2023**, *118*, 3272–3287. [CrossRef] [PubMed]
2. Blecker, S.; Paul, M.; Taksler, G.; Ogedegbe, G.; Katz, S. Heart failure–associated hospitalizations in the United States. *J. Am. Coll. Cardiol.* **2013**, *61*, 1259–1267. [CrossRef] [PubMed]
3. Biermann, J.; Neumann, T.; Angermann, C.E.; Erbel, R.; Maisch, B.; Pittrow, D.; Regitz-Zagrosek, V.; Scheffold, T.; Wachter, R.; Gelbrich, G.; et al. Economic burden of patients with various etiologies of chronic systolic heart failure analyzed by resource use and costs. *Int. J. Cardiol.* **2012**, *156*, 323–325. [CrossRef] [PubMed]
4. Heidenreich, P.A.; Albert, N.M.; Allen, L.A.; Bluemke, D.A.; Butler, J.; Fonarow, G.C.; Ikonomidis, J.S.; Khavjou, O.; Konstam, M.A.; Maddox, T.M.; et al. Forecasting the impact of heart failure in the United States: A policy statement from the American Heart Association. *Circ. Heart Fail* **2013**, *6*, 606–619. [CrossRef]
5. Wołowiec, Ł.; Rogowicz, D.; Banach, J.; Gilewski, W.; Sinkiewicz, W.; Grześk, G. Catestatin as a New Prognostic Marker in Stable Patients with Heart Failure with Reduced Ejection Fraction in Two-Year Follow-Up. *Dis. Markers* **2020**, *2020*, 8847211. [CrossRef]
6. Wołowiec, Ł.; Rogowicz, D.; Banach, J.; Buszko, K.; Surowiec, A.; Błażejewski, J.; Bujak, R.; Sinkiewicz, W. Prognostic significance of red cell distribution width and other red cell parameters in patients with chronic heart failure during two years of follow-up. *Kardiol. Pol.* **2016**, *74*, 657–664. [CrossRef]
7. Banach, J.; Grochowska, M.; Gackowska, L.; Buszko, K.; Bujak, R.; Gilewski, W.; Kubiszewska, I.; Wołowiec, Ł.; Michałkiewicz, J.; Sinkiewicz, W. Melanoma cell adhesion molecule as an emerging biomarker with prognostic significance in systolic heart failure. *Biomark. Med.* **2016**, *10*, 733–742. [CrossRef]
8. Banach, J.; Wołowiec, Ł.; Rogowicz, D.; Gackowska, L.; Kubiszewska, I.; Gilewski, W.; Michałkiewicz, J.; Sinkiewicz, W. Procalcitonin (PCT) Predicts Worse Outcome in Patients with Chronic Heart Failure with Reduced Ejection Fraction (HFrEF). *Dis. Markers* **2018**, *2018*, 9542784. [CrossRef] [PubMed]
9. Grześk, G.; Witczyńska, A.; Węglarz, M.; Wołowiec, Ł.; Nowaczyk, J.; Grześk, E.; Nowaczyk, A. Soluble Guanylyl Cyclase Activators-Promising Therapeutic Option in the Pharmacotherapy of Heart Failure and Pulmonary Hypertension. *Molecules* **2023**, *28*, 861. [CrossRef]
10. Woźniak-Wiśniewska, A.; Błażejewski, J.; Bujak, R.; Wołowiec, Ł.; Rogowicz, D.; Sinkiewicz, W. The value of cancer antigen 125 (Ca 125) and copeptin as markers in patients with advanced heart failure. *Folia Cardiol.* **2017**, *12*, 537–542. [CrossRef]
11. Rogowicz, D.; Wołowiec, Ł.; Banach, J.; Buszko, K.; Mosiądz, P.; Gilewski, W.; Zukow, W.; Sinkiewicz, W. Usefulness of serum high-sensitivity C-reactive protein (hs-CRP) level as prognostic factor in patients with chronic heart failure. *J. Educ. Health Sport* **2016**, *6*, 513–524. [CrossRef]
12. Pieroni, M.; Corti, A.; Tota, B.; Curnis, F.; Angelone, T.; Colombo, B.; Cerra, M.C.; Bellocci, F.; Crea, F.; Maseri, A. Myocardial production of chromogranin A in human heart: A new regulatory peptide of cardiac function. *Eur. Heart J.* **2007**, *28*, 1117. [CrossRef]
13. Biswas, N.; Curello, E.; O'Connor, D.T.; Mahata, S.K. Chromogranin/secretogranin proteins in murine heart: Myocardial production of chromogranin A fragment catestatin (Chga(364-384)). *Cell Tissue Res.* **2010**, *342*, 353–361. [CrossRef]
14. Liu, L.; Ding, W.; Li, R.; Ye, X.; Zhao, J.; Jiang, J.; Meng, L.; Wang, J.; Chu, S.; Han, X.; et al. Plasma levels and diagnostic value of catestatin in patients with heart failure. *Peptides* **2013**, *46*, 20–25. [CrossRef]
15. Mahata, S.K.; O'Connor, D.T.; Mahata, M.; Yoo, S.H.; Taupenot, L.; Wu, H.; Gill, B.M.; Parmer, R.J. Novel autocrine feedback control of catecholamine release. A discrete chromogranin a fragment is a noncompetitive nicotinic cholinergic antagonist. *J. Clin. Invest.* **1997**, *100*, 1623–1633. [CrossRef] [PubMed]
16. Mahata, S.K.; Mahata, M.; Wen, G.; Wong, W.B.; Mahapatra, N.R.; Hamilton, B.A.; O'Connor, D.T. The catecholamine release-inhibitory "catestatin" fragment of chromogranin a: Naturally occurring human variants with different potencies for multiple chromaffin cell nicotinic cholinergic responses. *Mol. Pharmacol.* **2004**, *66*, 1180–1191. [CrossRef] [PubMed]
17. Fung, M.M.; Salem, R.M.; Mehtani, P.; Thomas, B.; Lu, C.F.; Perez, B.; Rao, F.; Stridsberg, M.; Ziegler, M.G.; Mahata, S.K.; et al. Direct vasoactive effects of the chromogranin A (CHGA) peptide catestatin in humans in vivo. *Clin. Exp. Hypertens.* **2010**, *32*, 278–287. [CrossRef]
18. Røsjø, H.; Nygård, S.; Kaukonen, K.M.; Karlsson, S.; Stridsberg, M.; Ruokonen, E.; Pettilä, V.; Omland, T.; FINNSEPSIS Study Group. Prognostic value of chromogranin A in severe sepsis: Data from the FINNSEPSIS study. *Intensive Care Med.* **2012**, *38*, 820–829. [CrossRef] [PubMed]
19. Pei, Z.; Ma, D.; Ji, L.; Zhang, J.; Su, J.; Xue, W.; Chen, X.; Wang, W. Usefulness of catestatin to predict malignant arrhythmia in patients with acute myocardial infarction. *Peptides* **2014**, *55*, 131–135. [CrossRef]
20. Meng, L.; Ye, X.J.; Ding, W.H.; Yang, Y.; Di, B.B.; Liu, L.; Huo, Y. Plasma catecholamine release-inhibitory peptide catestatin in patients with essential hypertension. *J. Cardiovasc. Med.* **2011**, *12*, 643–647. [CrossRef]

21. Zalewska, E.; Kmieć, P.; Sworczak, K. Role of Catestatin in the Cardiovascular System and Metabolic Disorders. *Front. Cardiovasc. Med.* **2022**, *9*, 909480. [CrossRef]
22. Zhao, Y.; Zhu, D. Potential applications of catestatin in cardiovascular diseases. *Biomark. Med.* **2016**, *10*, 877–888. [CrossRef] [PubMed]
23. Liu, R.; Sun, N.L.; Yang, S.N.; Guo, J.Q. Catestatin could ameliorate proliferating changes of target organs in spontaneously hypertensive rats. *Chin. Med. J.* **2013**, *126*, 2157–2162. [PubMed]
24. Mazza, R.; Pasqua, T.; Gattuso, A. Cardiac heterometric response: The interplay between Catestatin and nitric oxide deciphered by the frog heart. *Nitric Oxide* **2012**, *27*, 40–49. [CrossRef] [PubMed]
25. Miyauchi, T.; Sakai, S. Endothelin and the heart in health and diseases. *Peptides* **2019**, *111*, 77–88. [CrossRef] [PubMed]
26. Pasqua, T.; Rocca, C.; Spena, A.; Angelone, T.; Cerra, M.C. Modulation of the coronary tone in the expanding scenario of Chromogranin-A and its derived peptides. *Future Med. Chem.* **2019**, *11*, 1501–1511. [CrossRef] [PubMed]
27. Chen, Y.; Wang, X.; Yang, C.; Su, X.; Yang, W.; Dai, Y.; Han, H.; Jiang, J.; Lu, L.; Wang, H.; et al. Decreased circulating catestatin levels are associated with coronary artery disease: The emerging anti-inflammatory role. *Atherosclerosis* **2019**, *281*, 78–88. [CrossRef]
28. Gallo, M.P.; Femminò, S.; Antoniotti, S.; Querio, G.; Alloatti, G.; Levi, R. Catestatin Induces Glucose Uptake and GLUT4 Trafficking in Adult Rat Cardiomyocytes. *Biomed Res. Int.* **2018**, *2018*, 2086109. [CrossRef]
29. Bandyopadhyay, G.; Tang, K.; Webster, N.J.G.; van den Bogaart, G.; Mahata, S.K. Catestatin induces glycogenesis by stimulating the phosphoinositide 3-kinase-AKT pathway. *Acta Physiol.* **2022**, *235*, e13775. [CrossRef]
30. Chu, S.Y.; Peng, F.; Wang, J.; Liu, L.; Meng, L.; Zhao, J.; Han, X.N.; Ding, W.H. Catestatin in defense of oxidative-stress-induced apoptosis: A novel mechanism by activating the beta2 adrenergic receptor and PKB/Akt pathway in ischemic-reperfused myocardium. *Peptides* **2020**, *123*, 170200. [CrossRef]
31. Ying, W.; Tang, K.; Avolio, E.; Schilling, J.M.; Pasqua, T.; Liu, M.A.; Cheng, H.; Gao, H.; Zhang, J.; Mahata, S.; et al. Immunosuppression of Macrophages Underlies the Cardioprotective Effects of CST (Catestatin). *Hypertension* **2021**, *77*, 1670–1682. [CrossRef]
32. Bandyopadhyay, G.K.; Vu, C.U.; Gentile, S.; Lee, H.; Biswas, N.; Chi, N.W.; O'Connor, D.T.; Mahata, S.K. Catestatin (chromogranin A(352-372) and novel effects on mobilization of fat from adipose tissue through regulation of adrenergic and leptin signaling. *J. Biol. Chem.* **2012**, *287*, 23141–23151. [CrossRef] [PubMed]
33. McDonagh, T.A.; Metra, M.; Adamo, M.; Adamo, M.; Gardner, R.S.; Baumbach, A.; Böhm, M.; Burri, H.; Butler, J.; Čelutkienė, J.; et al. 2021 ESC Guidelines for the diagnosis and treatment of acute and chronic heart failure. *Eur. Heart J.* **2021**, *42*, 3599–3726. [CrossRef] [PubMed]
34. Madamanchi, C.; Alhosaini, H.; Sumida, A.; Runge, M.S. Obesity and natriuretic peptides, BNP and nt-probnp: Mechanisms and diagnostic implications for heart failure. *Int. J. Cardiol.* **2014**, *176*, 611–617. [CrossRef]
35. Zhu, D.; Wang, F.; Yu, H.; Mi, L.; Gao, W. Catestatin is useful in detecting patients with stage B heart failure. *Biomarkers* **2011**, *16*, 691–697. [CrossRef]
36. Peng, F.; Chu, S.; Ding, W.; Liu, L.; Zhao, J.; Cui, X.; Li, R.; Wang, J. The predictive value of plasma catestatin for all-cause and cardiac deaths in chronic heart failure patients. *Peptides* **2016**, *86*, 112–117. [CrossRef]
37. Borovac, J.A.; Glavas, D.; Susilovic Grabovac, Z.; Supe Domic, D.; D'Amario, D.; Bozic, J. Catestatin in Acutely Decompensated Heart Failure Patients: Insights from the CATSTAT-HF Study. *J. Clin. Med.* **2019**, *8*, 1132. [CrossRef]
38. Grześk, G.; Wołowiec, Ł.; Rogowicz, D.; Gilewski, W.; Kowalkowska, M.; Banach, J.; Hertmanowski, W.; Dobosiewicz, M. The Importance of Pharmacokinetics, Pharmacodynamic and Repetitive Use of Levosimendan. *Biomed. Pharmacother.* **2022**, *153*, 113391. [CrossRef]
39. Grześk, G.; Dorota, B.; Wołowiec, Ł.; Wołowiec, A.; Osiak, J.; Kozakiewicz, M.; Banach, J. Safety of PCSK9 Inhibitors. *Biomed. Pharmacother.* **2022**, *156*, 113957. [CrossRef] [PubMed]

Disclaimer/Publisher's Note: The statements, opinions and data contained in all publications are solely those of the individual author(s) and contributor(s) and not of MDPI and/or the editor(s). MDPI and/or the editor(s) disclaim responsibility for any injury to people or property resulting from any ideas, methods, instructions or products referred to in the content.

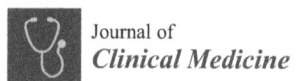

Review

Stress and Heart in Remodeling Process: Multiple Stressors at the Same Time Kill

Fatih Yalçin [1,2,*], Maria Roselle Abraham [1] and Mario J. Garcia [3]

1. Department of Cardiology, UCSF HEALTH, School of Medicine, Cardiac Imaging, San Francisco, CA 94143, USA; roselle.abraham@ucsf.edu
2. Department of Medicine, University of California at San Francisco, Cardiology UCSF Health, 505 Parnassus Avenue, Rm M314AUCSF, P.O. Box 0214, San Francisco, CA 94117, USA
3. Department of Cardiology, Montefiore Medical Center, Albert Einstein College of Medicine, Bronx, NY 10461, USA; mariogar@montefiore.org
* Correspondence: faith.yalcin@ucsf.edu

Abstract: Myocardial remodeling is developed by increased stress in acute or chronic pathophysiologies. Stressed heart morphology (SHM) is a new description representing basal septal hypertrophy (BSH) caused by emotional stress and chronic stress due to increased afterload in hypertension. Acute stress cardiomyopathy (ASC) and hypertension could be together in clinical practice. Therefore, there are some geometric and functional aspects regarding this specific location, septal base under acute and chronic stress stimuli. The findings by our and the other research groups support that hypertension-mediated myocardial involvement could be pre-existed in ASC cases. Beyond a frequently seen predominant base, hyperkinetic tissue response is detected in both hypertension and ASC. Furthermore, hypertension is the responsible factor in recurrent ASC. The most supportive prospective finding is BSH in which a hypercontractile base takes a longer time to exist morphologically than an acutely developed syndrome under both physiologic exercise and pressure overload by transaortic binding in small animals using microimaging. However, cardiac decompensation with apical ballooning could mask the possible underlying hypertensive disease. In fact, enough time for the assessment of previous hypertension history or segmental analysis could not be provided in an emergency unit, since ASC is accepted as an acute coronary syndrome during an acute episode. Additional supportive findings for SHM are increased stress scores in hypertensive BSH and the existence of similar tissue aspects in excessive sympathetic overdrive like pheochromocytoma which could result in both hypertensive disease and ASC. Exercise hypertension as the typical form of blood pressure variability is the sum of physiologic exercise and pathologic increased blood pressure and results in increased mortality. Hypertension is not rare in patients with a high stress score and leads to repetitive attacks in ASC supporting the important role of an emotional component as well as the potential danger due to multiple stressors at the same time. In the current review, the impact of multiple stressors on segmental or global myocardial remodeling and the hazardous potential of multiple stressors at the same time are discussed. As a result, incidentally determined segmental remodeling could be recalled in patients with multiple stressors and contribute to the early and combined management of both hypertension and chronic stress in the prevention of global remodeling and heart failure.

Keywords: hypertension; exercise hypertension; myocardial remodeling; autonomic nervous system; emotional stress; stress score; basal septal hypertrophy; stressed heart morphology; acute stress cardiomyopathy; heart failure

Citation: Yalçin, F.; Abraham, M.R.; Garcia, M.J. Stress and Heart in Remodeling Process: Multiple Stressors at the Same Time Kill. *J. Clin. Med.* **2024**, *13*, 2597. https://doi.org/10.3390/jcm13092597

Academic Editors: Francesco Pelliccia and Teruhiko Imamura

Received: 13 March 2024
Revised: 22 April 2024
Accepted: 24 April 2024
Published: 28 April 2024

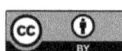

Copyright: © 2024 by the authors. Licensee MDPI, Basel, Switzerland. This article is an open access article distributed under the terms and conditions of the Creative Commons Attribution (CC BY) license (https://creativecommons.org/licenses/by/4.0/).

1. Introduction

In the cardiovascular disease continuum, short-term or long-term stress induction could possibly result in a variety of pathophysiological scenarios and clinical presentations.

Although the types of stressors may be different, myocardial tissue may have some specific morphologic and functional aspects [1–3]. It has been pointed out that acute myocardial infarction results in earlier left ventricular (LV) dysfunction compared to chronic hypertension and normal aging [4]. However, we proposed a new paradigm suggesting that certain acute clinical presentations may develop on a chronic pathophysiological base [5,6]. Documentation of a pre-existing chronic base in hypertension-mediated pathophysiology in acutely developed stress-related heart diseases such as ASC could be difficult [6]. Early septal LV remodeling, namely, basal septal hypertrophy (BSH) is related to different stressors like exercise hypertension [1], emotional in acute stress cardiomyopathy (ASC), [2,5,6], functional in hypertension-mediated increased afterload [7], and mechanical in aortic stenosis [8]. We validated BSH as the early imaging biomarker and described stressed heart morphology (SHM) as the specific location for superposed multiple stressors [9].

Since segmental remodeling is not generally used as a method in cardiac imaging, SHM could be underestimated in clinical practice despite it being a mutual finding in both hypertensive heart disease and ASC [5–7]. Hypertension is the most common killer in the population, however, approximately half of the total hypertensives stay undiagnosed, according to the World Health Organization [10]. Hypertension in the majority of clinical cases is associated with anxiety, depression, and panic attacks [11]. In our animal validation study, microimaging showed that physiologic and pathologic stressors lead to a very regularly progressed BSH (Figure 1a,b) differently from human beings [12–14]. In fact, we have focused on the psychological background in hypertensives with high stress scores who have shown extremely complex, irregular BSH with a myocardial tissue heterogeneity [9,15,16]. This was the main reason for us to describe SHM as the consequence of superposed multiple stressors. Selye began to employ a new term, "stressor" to differentiate between the harmful agent and the biological response more clearly: All agents can act as stressors, producing both stress and specific actions which could lead to some mechanisms including defense or damage in the tissues [17].

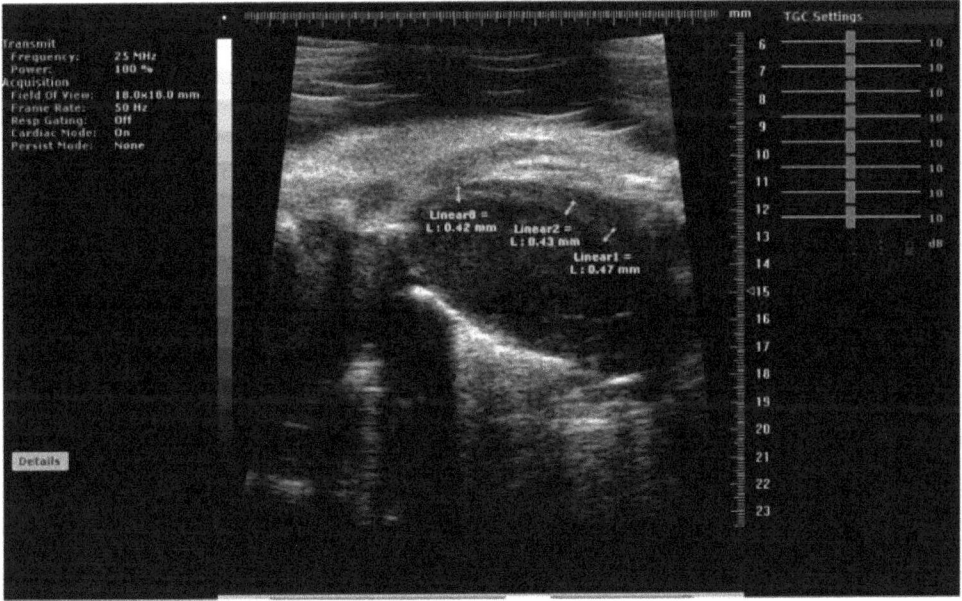

(a)

Figure 1. *Cont.*

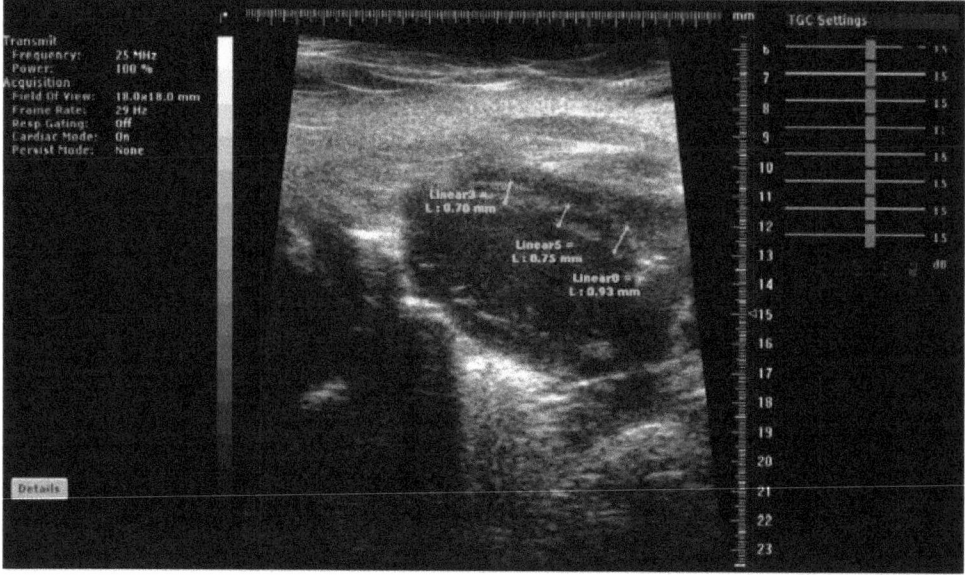

(b)

Figure 1. (a,b) Cardiac images of mice using 3rd-generation microscopic ultrasound show normal cardiac geometry and a regularly remodeled septal wall with thicker septal base at 4 weeks after stress induction due to pressure overload (TAC: transverse aortic construction), respectively.

Sympathetic innervation is the main factor for cardiac adaptation and LV remodeling under pressure overload and hemodynamic stress [18]. Histological abundance of post-ganglionic sympathetic neurons is a well-documented explanation for a locally dominant sympathetic overdrive which could be a possible mechanism for the role of a sympathetic drive in BSH [19,20]. The correlation between the autonomous nervous system and hypertension which is an absolute and documented risk factor for recurrent ASC [21] is commonly associated with emotional stress [17].

2. Chronic Stress

Stress is associated with both the psychological state and the physiological response of the body which can lead to anxiety and depression, as well as high blood pressure [11]. Therefore, hypertensive subjects could be facing severe emotional problems and develop a predominant septal base prior to acute episodic clinical presentations. In fact, episodic ASC could be an LV dysfunction due to both hypertension [21] and chronic stress as we have recently emphasized [6]. A variety of stressors such as exercise hypertension (Figure 2a–c) could be superposed over the LV septal base which is the unique part of a heart tissue free from parasympathetic modulation [9].

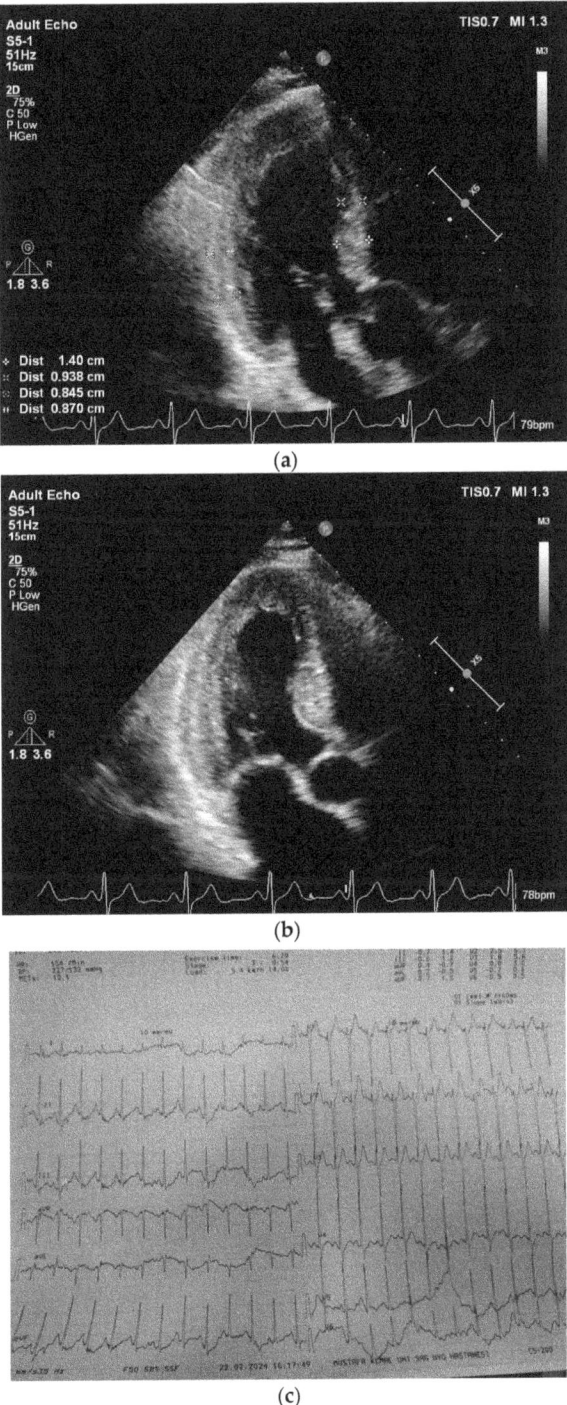

Figure 2. A slight curve of interventricular septal base from apical 4 chamber view during end-diastole (**a**) and end-systole (**b**) in a patient with exercise hypertension (a greater blood pressure response than 210/110 mmHg to peak exercise stress), (**c**) and basal septal hypertrophy.

3. Stress and Brain

Chronic stress could be more important than we think and preparing a base for the future acute episodic attacks as Dr. Ratey JJ. has pointed out, chronic stress is a threat to the body's balance and can tear at the architecture of the brain [11]. Additionally, he also emphasizes that emotions may not be separated by biological aspects. Furthermore, he describes that anything which activates the brain's cellular activity is a form of stress for the brain and the body. It looks difficult to separate emotions and relevant chronic cognitive abnormalities in human beings from blood pressure regulation pathways as well as hypertensive LV remodeling which is basically related to the sympathetic overdrive [5,6,9]. For the brain tissue, it was pointed out that plenty of activity is formulated by body movements which activates the specific neuronal signaling pathways between the body and the brain and these interactions produce emotions [11].

In fact, emotional reactions are associated with the general response of brain cellular activity under stress and could prepare a base with repetitive chronic stress, especially in the individuals with high stress scores prior to the acutely developed stress-induced syndromes [6]. Over the past years, there is increasing evidence about the brain–heart interaction with major potential implications for the treatment of cardiovascular diseases. Cerebrovascular accidents and transient ischemic attacks are frequently caused by hypertension and cardiac arrhythmias [11,22]. Brain architecture could be harmed by heart problems even in the absence of manifest stroke and atrial fibrillation is a risk factor for cognitive impairment and hippocampal atrophy [22,23]. Cognition and measures of structural brain integrity are important in cardiovascular problems. Panic disorders and emotional distress such as ASC may give rise to tachyarrhythmias with ensuing transient LV dysfunction [24]. We recently have pointed out that chronic stress-mediated SHM as a validated early imaging biomarker possibly plays a pre-existing role and prepares a base for acute emotional episodes [5–7,9,14–16].

4. Stress and Heart

We proposed that the complex septal base, SHM, is the specific conjunctive point of determination in a variety of stressors and represents the adaptive phase of LV remodeling [25]. SHM could take a dominant role as the early imaging biomarker in the management of multiple stressors at the same time in the near future. SHM could be more important than we think because it represents not only a specific morphologic aspect but some functional tissue aspects. Interestingly, cardiac response to stress like the brain tissue is related to cellular activity as we have published some clinical reports showing hyperdynamic myocardial response using fluid and tissue dynamics to stress induction [2,26–28]. Tissue adaptation independent from the type of stress has been generally accepted as a defense mechanism that uses accumulated energy. However, maladaptation of tissue to chronic stress is possibly related to the terminal phase with diminished cellular activity and accumulated energy which is generally accepted as the tissue damage phase [7,17,25].

Like the relation between a variety of body movements and the emotional response of the brain tissue [11], cardiovascular findings and emotions are also related [15–17,21–24]. While chronic cardiovascular disease progression has a complicated and multifactorial transaction including a genetic aspect, some potential missing links could possibly exist between chronic risk factors and sudden attacks like acute coronary syndrome (half of them may not be explained by classical risk factors) or ASC [1–3,5–7,14–16]. Beyond stress mechanics affected by systemic neurohormonal activation [17,29], sympathetic nerve activity could have an additional role [18–20].

5. Updated Knowledge for Superposed Multiple Stressors

1. SHM could have some specific geometric and functional aspects affected by a variety of stress stimuli or superposed multiple stressors [9,14–16].
2. Segmental remodeling, namely, SHM could be implemented in a clinical protocol for monitoring previously undiagnosed hypertension and increased stress [9,30–32].

3. The effect of superposed multiple stressors is independent from the type of stress and complex SHM with tissue heterogeneity in human beings (Figure 3a–c) having a striking difference from the regular segmental remodeling progression in small animals under stress induction determined by microimaging [12–14].

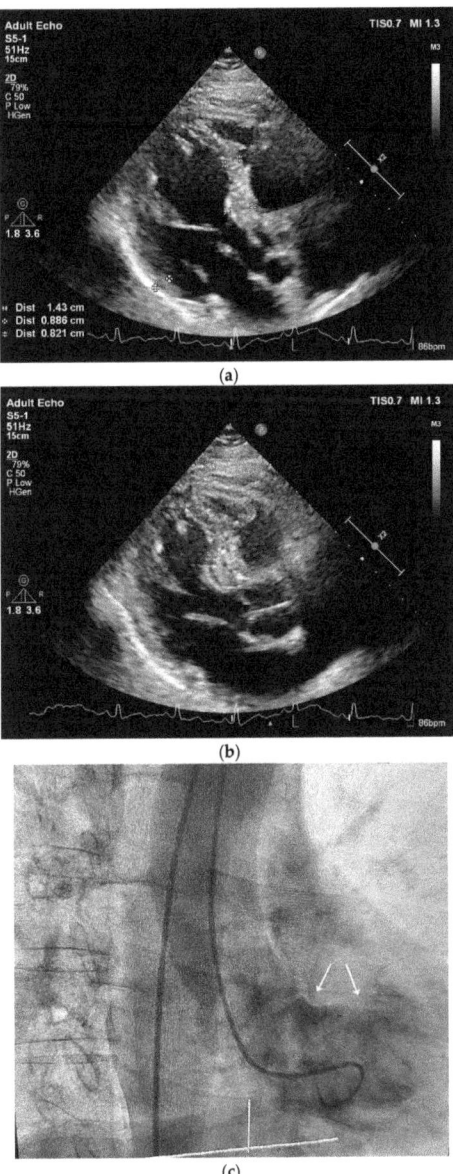

Figure 3. (a) Predominantly placed hypertrophy over septal base from apical 4 chamber view during end-diastole in a previously undiagnosed hypertensive patient with SHM who has undergone a recent earthquake and lost his two children during catastrophy. (b) A remarkable protruding basal septum with myocardial tissue heterogeneity into the LV cavity during systole in the same patient with a high level of stress score. (c) A remarkable basal cavity narrowing (pointed with white arrows), "Tako-tsubo like cardiac geometry" due to basal septal hypertrophy of the same patient in ventriculography.

4. Segmental LV remodeling instead of cross-sectional measurements could contribute to the prediction of future global LV remodeling and heart failure development due to basal apical discordance as we have recently proposed in patients with mechanic stress in aortic stenosis and functional stress in hypertension due to increased afterload, respectively [25,30–32].
5. The dominant role of the type of stress is not known in SHM, since there is a lack of the pooled data regarding segmental remodeling around the world as we recently have pointed out in our editorial [31].
6. There is a need to work on cell biology to search cellular levels of myocardial tissue to prove SHM as the specific location of Selye's theory on nonspecific general adaptive responses to stressors [17].
7. Importantly, literature data showing that intermittent adrenergic stimulation [33] in animal models is more dangerous than static sympathetic stimulation in terms of LV remodeling development (Scheme 1).

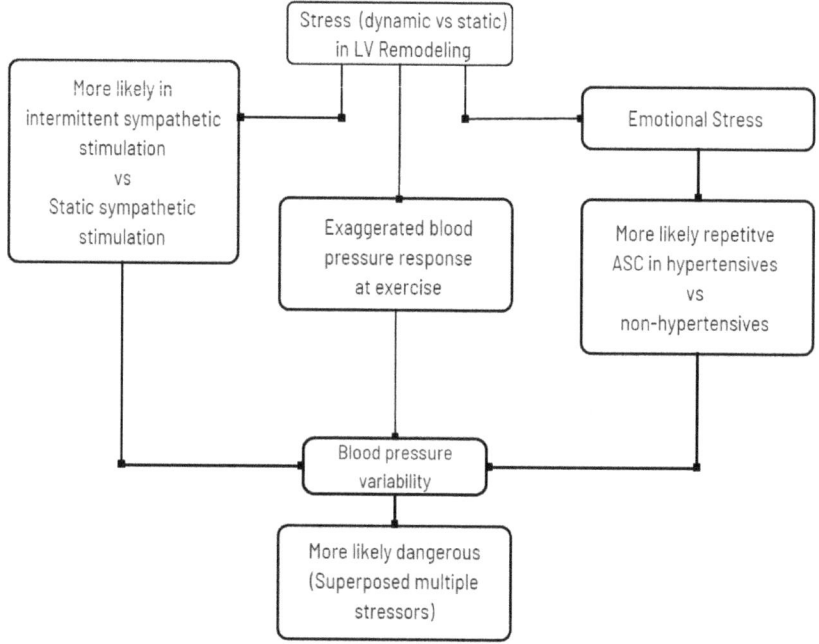

Scheme 1. The hazardous effect of superposed multiple stressors.

8. We pointed out the importance of stress-induced exaggerated hypertension and hemodynamic overload under stress in the patients with BSH [1,15,25]. Years later, we realized the importance of emotional factors on very complex BSH [2,5–7,15,16,31] after we validated BSH as the early imaging biomarker during very regular LV remodeling in small animals using 3rd-generation microscopic ultrasonography [12–14].
9. In addition to increased stress scores and more cognitive problems in hypertensives [6,15,16] compared to non-hypertensives, it was shown that recurrent ASC is more commonly detected in hypertensive patients possibly due to hemodynamic fluctuations [21,34]. Long-term variability in blood pressure is now known to be related to increased mortality than the effect of mean blood pressure [35,36].
10. In addition to its relation to SHM, superposed multiple stressors including increased adrenergic overdrive [9,21,34], cognitive disorders [6,15,16], chronic or exercise hypertension [1], which are also associated with increased cardiovascular mortality [37,38], are more likely dangerous since each risk is associated with LV remodeling with

hemodynamic overload [1,2,5–9,25–28] and represents hemodynamic fluctuations due to blood pressure variability which is associated with increased mortality [35,36].

6. Future Perspective

Hypertension could possibly be the case prior to the first ASC episode since recurrent ASC attacks relate to hypertension. Combined daily stressful components like exercise hypertension, emotional stress, or excessive sympathetic overdrive like pheochromocytoma result in hemodynamic overload with blood pressure variability that could be a potential killer like exercise hypertension and prevented by comprehensive neuro-cardiologic perspective. SHM should be recorded globally and evaluated more comprehensively since all stressful components could potentially be determined in SHM patients.

A variety of stressors could be superposed over the septal base as the specific location which is the unique human tissue free of parasympathetic modulation. Anxiety, depression, and panic attacks are not rare in hypertension. Since undiagnosed hypertensive heart disease has become more prevalent, we strongly suggest segmental evaluation instead of single cross-section and point out the importance and potential advantages of determination of echocardiographic segmental geometric data. Beyond pure hemodynamic overload, SHM does not spread over other myocardial segments (Figure 4) which is why combined assessment of the heart and brain will possibly have an additional advantage to preventing "the hazardous effect of superposed multiple stressors" (Scheme 1).

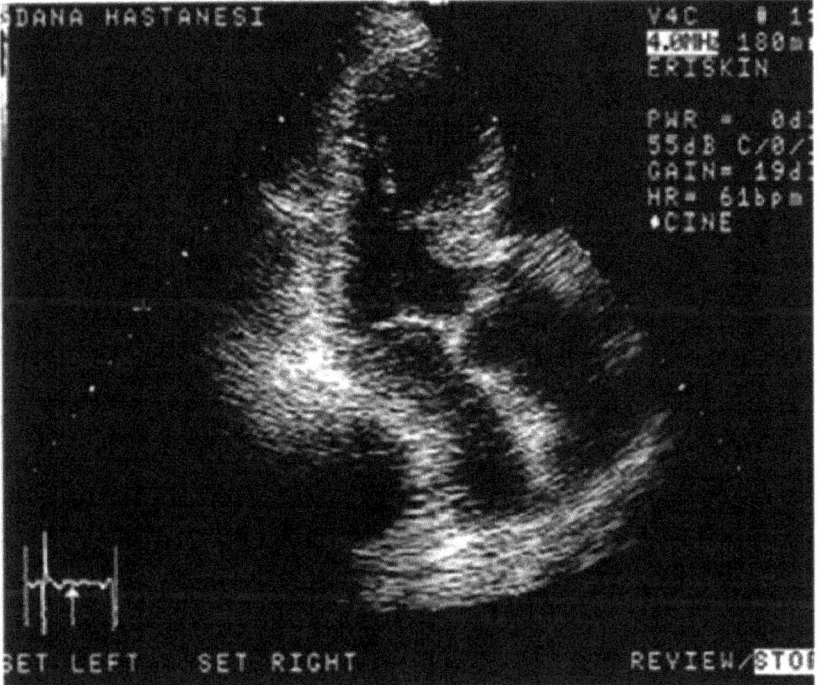

Figure 4. Enormously localized SHM over septal base in a hypertensive patient, a parliament representative with very high stress score [5,15].

Moreover, this new paradigm could be beneficial to explore missed cases with hypertension and to document whether or not these individuals have increased stress score prior to acute stress-related cardiac attacks. Sympathetic overdrive with palpitation, sweating, tremor, red face, etc., in pheochromocytoma could be the most typical presentation of superposed multiple stressors including hypertension and emotional stress. Episodic emotion-mediated hemodynamic fluctuation with blood pressure variability due to multiple stressors at the same time in humans is a consistent finding with the hazardous effect of intermittent sympathetic stimulation in animals.

Baroreflex sensitivity and heart rate variability are important parameters in the unique role of the autonomic nervous system on both the heart and brain. In fact, we detected that respiratory exercise has a special role in clinical practice which can provide an important benefit in the control of combined hypertension and emotional problems [39]. In addition to classic prevention using salt restriction and drugs, activity vagal stimulation, exercise training with blood pressure control, electrical neurostimulation, music therapy, and, recently, global assessment and management of hypertensive patients with high stress scores have become interesting topics.

7. Stress History

Adaptation to stressors independent from the type of stress is related to a systemic neurohormonal mechanism, namely, general adaptation syndrome [40]. Clinical features of disease could be the result of a failure in the nonspecific adaptive mechanisms of the body [41]. General adaptation syndrome was described by Selye and adrenal glands were shown as the critical organ that plays a central role in adaptive reactions [42]. Acute and prolonged overstimulation by physical or emotional trauma affects the body leading to the release of adrenaline and having a harmful effect on the previously balanced system in terms of function and geometry, as well as energetics [43].

Selye introduced a new term as stressor which describes both harmful agent and the biological response, therefore, all agents can act as stressors, producing both stress and specific actions [5]. Since there is difficulty in differentiating the harmful agent and the biological response, high technologic methods were used longstandingly, but certain separative formulas could not have become clinically practical. Selye also used a new notion as adaptation energy [43] in description of sufficient tolerance to different forms of injury, showing the stage of tissue resistance. He also mentioned the limited energy as eventual exhaustion and death due to repeated environmental stress [41]. Stress also was interpreted as the interaction between damage and defense or force and resistance which is completely similar to adaptive response to stress before tissue damage [17]. Stress is used practically as the common denominator of all adaptive reactions in the body and more specifically, stress, rather than adaptation, indicated the central biological course at the general and complex reactions in the body [17]. Stress acts not only as an external trigger of internal processes but as the physiological or pathological process itself [40].

Selye's attempt to develop a novel theoretical framework for understanding a range of biological reactions and clinical manifestations built up a base at the endocrinologic level, which is basically a neurohumoral response to external trauma describing nonspecific general adaptive response without any struggle to describe a specific location, function, or mechanism beyond a systemic response due to neurohumoral activation in circulation. Nevertheless, stress-related studies persist until much more experimental work has been conducted to separate specific physiological effects from those of a nonspecific nature [44]. Selye's studies of adaptation and stress were supported financially and the general adaptation syndrome constituted a philosophical point of view for disease concept. Those works were also evaluated by medical platforms and resulted in a new data pool of Bethesda regarding the new disease concept [45].

8. Autonomic Nervous System and Stressed Heart Findings

Neurologic perspective and modern neuroendocrinology were partly built up by the intellectual depth and remarkable energy in Selye's work on contemporary biology [46]. Stability in mental and emotional processes is possibly provided by the interactions of the body's subsystem interactions which needs a synchronization between the two branches of the autonomic nervous system (ANS) [47]. Sympathetic and parasympathetic activity in ANS with heart–brain synchronization contribute to the stability of the processes to maintain cardiovascular health with the regulation of heart rate, blood pressure at rest, and under physiologic and pathologic stress.

Balance of ANS is an important target to regulate for cardiovascular stability including the resetting of baroreceptor sensitivity, which is related to the improvement in short-term blood pressure control and increased respiratory efficiency. ANS balance also provides increased vagal afferent traffic, which is placed in the function of inhibiting pain signals and sympathetic outflow. In addition, ANS balance will contribute to the control of increased cardiac output with increased ability of the cardiovascular system to adapt to circulatory requirements [47]. After the importance of ANS in cardiovascular problems was understood clearly, new efforts and perspectives regarding increased cardiovascular risk factors like hypertension with emotional problems were started [39]. These efforts focus on the interrelation of multiple stressors different from the scientific efforts of Selye on the separation of physiological or pathological processes as the internal responses to external triggers or stressors [9].

In cardiovascular diseases, ASC, which is a clinical spectrum including emotional stress and related temporary LV dysfunction, seems to be the most typical phenomenon started by emotional instability [5]. In patients with ASC, an increased wall stress of acute emotional stress on the midapical part as the pathophysiologic mechanism leads to an episodic decompensation [6]. The regional LV base is relatively more resistant to stress compared to the midapical region in this phenomenon and is associated with a hyperdynamic aspect under emotional stress [5]. Similarly, hyperdynamic basal tissue with focal basal hypertrophy is also the case in hypertensive patients [26]. In the chronic period, episodic stress induces the heart to give a response of high heart rate-pressure product and high LV outflow tract blood flow, as well as basal septal hyperdynamic tissue in BSH patients with hypertension [27].

We described SHM because the predominant LV base with adaptive hypercontractility and a relatively larger midapical cavity is a conjunctive point of determination in clinical conditions, not only with chronic stress due to increased afterload in hypertension but with acute emotional stress in ASC [2,5]. These clinic observations possibly represented a compensatory segmental adaptation to increased stress stimuli in this group of patients. Beyond these cross-sectional observations, we decided to determine the progression of LV segmental remodeling prospectively. We used treadmill exercise for physiologic and transaortic construction for pathologic stress stimuli and 3rd-generation microscopic ultrasonography in the small animals for the determination of segmental LV remodeling evolution. In this study, we noted for the first time that BSH is the early imaging biomarker of LV remodeling under both physiologic and pathologic stress [12,13]. Nevertheless, since we detected BSH development as the initial LV remodeling prospectively in animal models in both physiologic stress-mediated remodeling with normal organization of myocytes and pathologic with myocyte hypertrophy and collagen accumulation, correct diagnosis for the nature of human BSH should be documented by blood pressure monitorization to explore whether or not pressure overload is the case in clinical practice [1–3].

We believe that these segmental aspects of LV under stress are important in a variety of clinical conditions with acute or chronic stress [5–7]. Animal validation studies years later than our description of SHM provided an understanding of the effect of high stress scores on the complex morphology over BSH in human beings differently from regular segmental remodeling in animal models under pathologic stress due to pressure overload [14–16]. Beyond emotional etiology, we mention the morphologic importance of segmental LV remodeling in stress-related cardiovascular diseases including mechanical stress due to aortic stenosis which is associated with SHM [8,32].

9. Nonspecific Stress Adaptation of Selye and Segmental Remodeling

Furthermore, it could be extremely difficult to find the dominant type of stress-shaping complex SHM in humans with exercise hypertension which has combined physiologic and pathologic stress. Except for the emotional component, both pressure overload as pathologic and treadmill exercise as physiologic stress in animals represent human exercise hypertension in the real world [14–16]. In this new paradigm, a complex heart base signifies the importance of cognitive function in humans [9]. Hypersensitivity of this special tissue to multiple stressors which could be superposed over the heart base could be a substrate for further research to explore whether this finding has a specific role in the adaptive process under nonspecific external stressors which are independent of acute, chronic, or focal neurohumoral response in myocardial tissue or systemic neurohumoral response as hypothesized by Hans Selye [17,40–43].

While blood pressure variability or exaggerated blood pressure response to exercise is important cardiovascular risks, improvement in both emotional and hemodynamic balance with blood pressure stability can contribute to cardiovascular health. This mode is associated with reduced perceptions of stress, sustained positive affect, and a high degree of mental clarity and emotional stability. We noted in hypertensives that specific rhythmic breathing methods may induce heart rhythm coherence and stability of increased blood pressure and depression [39].

In the respiratory–sympathetic connection with hypertension, the respiratory and circulatory systems are both involved in the delivery of oxygen and removal of carbon dioxide in the tissues [48]. Any alteration in this connection could result in cardiovascular consequences. Indeed, it was observed that this connection could lead to an increase in respiratory modulation of sympathetic overdrive that possibly contributes to the development of hypertension [49]. Both healthy and active people can experience a variety of limitations due to weak respiratory muscles. An increased respiratory–sympathetic connection may be responsible for the difficulty in the management of hypertension in humans [48,49].

In fact, studies have demonstrated that the strength of the inspiratory muscle plays a crucial role in the pathophysiology of exercise limitation in a variety of clinical disorders [50]. Inspiratory muscle weakness was detected in hypertension, one of the increasingly common risk factors and exercise capacity was negatively affected by this weakness [51]. Research studies on respiratory exercises that effects exercise capacity, one of the alternative treatments of hypertension, recently have been gaining importance. Ublosakka-Jones et al. [52] found that respiratory exercise training given at a low load for 8 weeks was effective on arm endurance capacity. An improvement in respiratory performance capacity caused by muscle endurance training in normotensive elderly patients continued with prolonged active training for 5 weeks [53]. It was observed that an 8-week workload applied to the inspiratory muscles can increase exercise capacity [54]. It is known that individual quality of life with hypertension is worse than normotensive individuals [55].

Breathing control is beneficial in lowering blood pressure in hypertension patients [56]. Respiratory exercises are beneficial due to ANS which impacts physiological respiration, emotion, and cognition mechanisms [57]. These exercises reduce sympathetic nervous system activity while enhancing parasympathetic nervous system activity, linked to cardiac vagal tone. Consequently, these exercises influence emotions, emotional regulation, psychological adaptation, reactivity, expression, and empathic responses. Utilizing this mechanism, breathing exercises can potentially be beneficial for conditions like depression [57].

We observed that device-assisted respiratory exercises performed with or without a certain workload yielded a benefit in the severity of depression in hypertension patients [40]. In our study examining the effect of inspiratory muscle training on quality of life in patients with hypertension, we observed that 8 weeks of breathing exercises training, including whether unloaded, low load intensity, or high load intensity training, decreased resting blood pressure in hypertension patients [39]. Breathing exercises and cardiovascular modulation work are crucial components of maintaining cardiovascular homeostasis and respiratory training is an effective method in the effective control of blood pressure [58].

Evaluation of hypertensives with a combined antihypertensive approach and stress management under a neurocardiologic perspective with comprehensive diagnostic tests are unmet needs in current clinical practice. We noted that incidentally determined segmental

LV remodeling and basal septal hypertrophy using basal and midapical measurements are crucial, instead of a single cross-sectional measurement on the cardiovascular imaging. Specific tissue aspects of SHM could be implemented in a practical clinical protocol not only for previously undiagnosed hypertension but cognitive disorders in clinical practice.

SHM should also be implemented in a practical clinical protocol for monitoring future acute episodes due to hypertension. Evaluation of hypertensives with a combined antihypertensive approach and stress management under a new neurocardiologic perspective with comprehensive diagnostic tests are currently unmet needs. In conclusion, incidentally determined segmental LV remodeling, namely, SHM, could be recorded during clinical practice globally and evaluated more comprehensively [9]. Beyond the clinical aspect of SHM, there is a need to focus on cell biology to work on cellular levels of myocardial tissue to search whether SHM is the specific location of Selye's nonspecific general adaptive response to stressors.

Funding: This research received no internal or external funding.

Acknowledgments: F.Y. is supported by the US Government Fulbright Scholarship, Washington DC, USA. He has accepted only research equipment support from Novartis Pharmaceuticals.

Conflicts of Interest: The authors declare no conflicts of interest.

Abbreviations

SHM	stressed heart morphology
BSH	basal septal hypertrophy
ASC	acute stress cardiomyopathy
LV	left ventricular
ANS	autonomic nervous system

References

1. Yalçin, F.; Yalçin, H.; Abraham, T.P. Exercise hypertension should be recalled in basal septal hypertrophy as the early imaging biomarker in patients with stressed heart morphology. *Blood Press. Monit.* **2020**, *25*, 118–119. [CrossRef] [PubMed]
2. Yalçin, F.; Yalçin, H.; Abraham, T. Stress-induced regional features of left ventricle is related to pathogenesis of clinical conditions with both acute and chronic stress. *Int. J. Cardiol.* **2010**, *145*, 367–368. [CrossRef] [PubMed]
3. Yalçin, F.; Topaloglu, C.; Kuçukler, N.; Ofgeli, M.; Abraham, T.P. Could early septal involvement in the remodeling process be related to the advance hypertensive heart disease? *Int. J. Cardiol. Heart Vasc.* **2015**, *7*, 141–145. [CrossRef] [PubMed]
4. Wang, J.; Fang, F.; Yip, G.W.-K.; Sanderson, J.E.; Feng, W.; Xie, J.-M.; Luo, X.-X.; Lee, A.P.-W.; Lam, Y.-Y. Left ventricular long-axis performance during exercise is an important prognosticator in patients with heart failure and preserved ejection fraction. *Int. J. Cardiol.* **2015**, *178*, 131–135. [CrossRef] [PubMed]
5. Yalçin, F.; Muderrisoğlu, H. Tako-tsubo cardiomyopathy may be associated with cardiac geometric features as observed in hypertensive heart disease. *Int. J. Cardiol.* **2009**, *135*, 251–252. [CrossRef] [PubMed]
6. Yalçin, F.; Çağatay, B.; Küçükler, N.; Abraham, T.P. Geomeric and functional aspects in hypertension and takotsubo: Importance of basal septal hypertrophy. *Eur. J. Prev. Cardiol.* **2023**, *30*, 1996–1997. [CrossRef] [PubMed]
7. Yalçin, F.; Yalçin, H.; Abraham, M.R.; Abraham, T.P. Ultimate phases of hypertensive heart disease and stressed heart morphology by conventional and novel cardiac imaging. *Am. J. Cardiovasc. Dis.* **2021**, *11*, 628–634. [PubMed]
8. Yalçin, F.; Abraham, R.; Abraham, T.P. Myocardial Aspects in Aortic Stenosis and Functional Increased Afterload Conditions in Patients with Stressed Heart Morphology. *Ann. Thorac. Cardiovasc. Surg.* **2021**, *27*, 332–334. [CrossRef]
9. Yalçin, F. *Stressed Heart Morphology: Specific Finding for Superposed Multiple Stressors*, 1st ed.; Yalçin, F., Ed.; Klinikleri: Ankara, Türkiye, 2022.
10. NCD Risk Factor Collaboration (NCD-RisC). Worldwide trends in hypertension prevalence and progress in treatment and control from 1990 to 2019: A pooled analysis of 1201 population-representative studies with 104 million participants. *Lancet* **2021**, *398*, 957–980. [CrossRef]
11. Ratey, J.; Hagerman, E. *Spark: The Revolutionary New Science of Exercise and the Brain*; Little, Brown Spark: New York, NY, USA, 2008; Volume 59.
12. Yalçin, F.; Kucukler, N.; Cingolani, O.H.; Mbiyangandu, B.; Sorensen, L.; Pinherio, A.; Abraham, M.R.; Abraham, T.P. Evolution of ventricular hypertrophy and myocardial mechanics in physiological and pathological hypertrophy. *J. Appl. Physiol.* **2019**, *126*, 354–362. [CrossRef]

13. Yalcin, F.; Kucukler, N.; Cingolani, O.; Mbiyangandu, B.; Sorensen, L.L.; Pinheiro, A.C.; Abraham, M.R.; Abraham, T.P. Intracavitary gradients in mice with early regional remodeling at the compensatory hyperactive stage prior to lv tissue dysfunction. *J. Am. Coll. Cardiol.* **2020**, *75*, 1585. [CrossRef]
14. Yalçin, F.; Yalçin, H.; Abraham, R.; Abraham, T.P. Hemodynamic stress and microscopic remodeling. *Int. J. Cardiol. Cardiovasc. Risk Prev.* **2021**, *11*, 200115. [CrossRef] [PubMed]
15. Yalçin, F.; Abraham, R.; Abraham, T.P. Basal septal hypertrophy: Extremely sensitive region to variety of stress stimuli and stressed heart morphology. *J. Hypertens.* **2022**, *40*, 626–627. [CrossRef]
16. Yalcin, F.; Melek, I.; Mutlu, T. Stressed heart morphology and neurologic stress core effect beyond hemodynamic stress on focal geometry. *J. Hypertens.* **2022**, *40*, e79.
17. Selye, H. *The Stress of Life*; McGraw-Hill: New York, NY, USA, 1956.
18. Schlaich, M.P.; Kaye, D.M.; Lambert, E.; Sommerville, M.; Socratous, F.; Esler, M.D. Relation between cardiac sympathetic activity and hypertensive left ventricular hypertrophy. *Circulation* **2003**, *108*, 560–565. [CrossRef] [PubMed]
19. Holmgren, S.; Abrahamsson, T.; Almgren, O. Adrenergic innervation of coronary arteries and ventricular myocardium in the pig: Fluorescence microscopic appearance in the normal state and after ischemia. *Basic. Res. Cardiol.* **1985**, *80*, 18–26. [CrossRef]
20. Kawano, H.; Okada, R.; Yano, K. Histological study on the distribution of autonomic nerves in the human heart. *Heart Vessel.* **2003**, *18*, 32–39. [CrossRef]
21. Liang, J.; Zhang, J.; Xu, Y.; Teng, C.; Lu, X.; Wang, Y.; Zuo, X.; Li, Q.; Huang, Z.; Ma, J.; et al. Conventional cardiovascular risk factors associated with Takotsubo cardiomyopathy: A comprehensive review. *Clin. Cardiol.* **2021**, *44*, 1033–1040. [CrossRef]
22. Osteraas, N.D.; Lee, V.H. Chapter 4—Neurocardiology. In *Critical Care Neurology Part I*; Handbook of Clinical Neurology; Wijdicks, E.F.M., Kramer, A.H., Eds.; Elsevier: Amsterdam, The Netherlands, 2017; Volume 140, pp. 49–65.
23. Taggart, P. Brain-heart interactions and cardiac ventricular arrhythmias. *Neth. Heart J.* **2012**, *21*, 78–81. [CrossRef]
24. Frommeyer, G.; Eckardt, L.; Breithardt, G. Panic attacks and supraventricular tachycardias: The chicken or the egg? *Neth. Heart J.* **2013**, *21*, 74–77. [CrossRef]
25. Yalçin, F.; Yalçin, H.; Küçükler, N.; Arslan, S.; Akkuş, O.; Kurtul, A.; Abraham, M.R. Basal Septal Hypertrophy as the Early Imaging Biomarker for Adaptive Phase of Remodeling Prior to Heart Failure. *J. Clin. Med.* **2021**, *11*, 75. [CrossRef] [PubMed]
26. Yalçin, F.; Yiğit, F.; Erol, T.; Baltali, M.; Korkmaz, M.E.; Müderrisoğlu, H. Effect of dobutamine stress on basal septal tissue dynamics in hypertensive patients with basal septal hypertrophy. *J. Hum. Hypertens.* **2006**, *20*, 628–630. [CrossRef] [PubMed]
27. Yalçin, F.; Muderrisoglu, H.; Korkmaz, M.E.; Ozin, B.; Baltali, M.; Yigit, F. The effect of dobutamine stress on left ventricular outflow tract gradients in hypertensive patients with basal septal hypertrophy. *Angiology* **2004**, *55*, 295–301. [CrossRef] [PubMed]
28. Yalçin, F.; Schindler, T.; Abraham, T.P. Hypertension should be ruled out in patients with hyperdynamic left ventricle on radionuclide myocardial perfusion imaging, diastolic dysfunction and dyspnea on exertion. *Int. J. Cardiol. Heart Vasc.* **2015**, *7*, 149–150. [CrossRef] [PubMed]
29. Wittstein, I.S.; Thiemann, D.R.; Lima, J.A.C.; Baughman, K.L.; Schulman, S.P.; Gerstenblith, G.; Wu, K.C.; Rade, J.J.; Bivalacqua, T.J.; Champion, H.C. Neurohumoral features of myocardial stunning due to sudden emotional stress. *N. Engl. J. Med.* **2005**, *352*, 539–548. [CrossRef] [PubMed]
30. Korhonen, P.E.; Kautiainen, H.; Järvenpää, S.; Kantola, I. Target organ damage and cardiovascular risk factors among subjects with previously undiagnosed hypertension. *Eur. J. Prev. Cardiol.* **2014**, *21*, 980–988. [CrossRef] [PubMed]
31. Yalcin, F.; Garcia, M.J. It is time to focus on "Segmental Remodeling" with validated biomarkers as "Stressed Heart Morphology" in prevention of heart failure. *J. Clin. Med.* **2022**, *11*, 4180. [CrossRef] [PubMed]
32. Yalçin, F.; Abraham, M.R.; Abraham, T.P. It is time to assess left ventricular segmental remodelling in aortic stenosis. *Eur. Heart J.-Cardiovasc. Imaging* **2022**, *23*, e299–e300. [CrossRef] [PubMed]
33. Werhahn, S.M.; Kreusser, J.S.; Hagenmüller, M.; Beckendorf, J.; Diemert, N.; Hoffmann, S.; Schultz, J.-H.; Backs, J.; Dewenter, M. Adaptive versus maladaptive cardiac remodelling in response to sustained β-adrenergic stimulation in a new "ISO on/off model". *PLoS ONE* **2021**, *16*, e0248933. [CrossRef]
34. Spes, C.; Knape, A.; Mudra, H. Recurrent tako–tsubo–like left ventricular dysfunction (apical ballooning) in a patient with pheochromocytoma—A case report. *Clin. Res. Cardiol.* **2006**, *95*, 307–311. [CrossRef]
35. Stevens, S.L.; Wood, S.; Koshiaris, C.; Law, K.; Glasziou, P.; Stevens, R.J.; McManus, R.J. Blood pressure variability and cardiovascular disease: Systematic review and meta-analysis. *BMJ* **2016**, *354*, i4098. [CrossRef]
36. Wang, J.; Shi, X.; Ma, C.; Zheng, H.; Xiao, J.; Bian, H.; Ma, Z.; Gong, L. Visit-to-visit blood pressure variability is a risk factor for all-cause mortality and cardiovascular disease: A systematic review and meta-analysis. *J. Hypertens.* **2017**, *35*, 10–17. [CrossRef] [PubMed]
37. Mundal, R.; Kjeldsen, S.E.; Sandvik, L.; Erikssen, G.; Thaulow, E.; Erikssen, J. Exercise blood pressure predicts mortality from myocardial infarction. *Hypertension* **1996**, *27*, 324–329. [CrossRef] [PubMed]
38. Schultz, M.G.; Otahal, P.; Cleland, V.J.; Blizzard, L.; Marwick, T.H.; Sharman, J.E. Exercise-induced hypertension, cardiovascular events, and mortality in patients undergoing exercise stress testing: A systematic review and meta-analysis. *Am. J. Hypertens.* **2013**, *26*, 357–366. [CrossRef] [PubMed]
39. Hüzmeli, I.; Katayifçi, N.; Yalçin, F.; Hüzmeli, E.D. Effects of different ınspiratory muscle training protocols on exercise capacity, respiratory muscle strength, and health-related quality of life in Patients with Hypertension. *Int. J. Clin. Pract.* **2024**, *2024*, 4136457. [CrossRef] [PubMed]

40. Selye, H. The general adaptation syndrome and the diseases of adaptation. *J. Clin. Endocrinol. Metab.* **1946**, *6*, 117–230. [CrossRef] [PubMed]
41. Selye, H. *The Story of the Adaptation Syndrome*; Aeta, Inc.: Montreal, QC, Canada, 1952; Volume 35.
42. Selye, H. The Significance of the Adrenals for Adaptation. *Science* **1937**, *85*, 247–248. [CrossRef] [PubMed]
43. Selye, H. Experimental evidence supporting the conception of "adaptation energy". *Am. J. Physiol. Content* **1938**, *123*, 758–765. [CrossRef]
44. Selye, H. Role of somatotrophic hormone in the production of malignant nephrosclerosis, periarteritis nodosa, and hypertensive disease. *Br. Med. J.* **1951**, *1*, 263–270. [CrossRef]
45. Selye, H. *Stress of My Life. 143. Illustration*; Rockefeller Foundation Archives, Rockefeller Archive Center, Sleepy Hollow: New York, NY, USA, 1950.
46. Cox, T. *Stress*; Macmillan: London, UK, 1978; p. 174.
47. Waxenbaum, J.A.; Reddy, V.; Varacallo, M. *Anatomy, Autonomic Nervous System*; StatPearls Publishing: Treasure Island, FL, USA, 2024.
48. Macefield, V. Finding inspiration in high blood pressure. *Exp. Physiol.* **2016**, *101*, 1449–1450. [CrossRef]
49. Simms, A.E.; Paton, J.F.R.; Pickering, A.E.; Allen, A.M. Amplified respiratory–sympathetic coupling in the spontaneously hypertensive rat: Does it contribute to hypertension? *J. Physiol.* **2009**, *587*, 597–610. [CrossRef] [PubMed]
50. Cipriano, G.F.; Cipriano, G.; Santos, F.V.; Güntzel Chiappa, A.M.; Pires, L.; Cahalin, L.P.; Chiappa, G.R. Current insights of inspiratory muscle training on the cardiovascular system: A systematic review with meta-analysis. *Integr. Blood Press. Control.* **2019**, *12*, 1–11. [CrossRef] [PubMed]
51. da Silva, C.D.; de Abreu, R.M.; Rehder-Santos, P.; De Noronha, M.; Catai, A.M. Can respiratory muscle training change the blood pressure levels in hypertension? A systematic review with meta-analysis. *Scand. J. Med. Sci. Sports* **2021**, *31*, 1384–1394. [CrossRef]
52. Ublosakka-Jones, C.; Tongdee, P.; Pachirat, O.; Jones, D.A. Slow loaded breathing training improves blood pressure, lung capacity and arm exercise endurance for older people with treated and stable isolated systolic hypertension. *Exp. Gerontol.* **2018**, *108*, 48–53. [CrossRef] [PubMed]
53. Stutz, J.; Casutt, S.; Spengler, C.M. Respiratory muscle endurance training improves exercise performance but does not affect resting blood pressure and sleep in healthy active elderly. *Eur. J. Appl. Physiol.* **2022**, *122*, 2515–2531. [CrossRef] [PubMed]
54. Wu, W.; Guan, L.; Zhang, X.; Li, X.; Yang, Y.; Guo, B.; Ou, Y.; Lin, L.; Zhou, L.; Chen, R. Effects of two types of equal-intensity inspiratory muscle training in stable patients with chronic obstructive pulmonary disease: A randomised controlled trial. *Respir. Med.* **2017**, *132*, 84–91. [CrossRef] [PubMed]
55. Trevisol, D.J.; Moreira, L.B.; Kerkhoff, A.; Fuchs, S.C.; Fuchs, F.D. Health-related quality of life and hypertension: A systematic review and meta-analysis of observational studies. *J. Hypertens.* **2011**, *29*, 179–188. [CrossRef] [PubMed]
56. Cheung, B.M.Y.; Lo, J.L.F.; Fong, D.Y.T.; Chan, M.Y.; Wong, S.H.T.; Wong, V.C.W.; Lam, K.S.L.; Lau, C.P.; Karlberg, J.P.E. Randomized controlled trial of qigong in the treatment of mild essential hypertension. *J. Hum. Hypertens.* **2005**, *19*, 697–704. [CrossRef] [PubMed]
57. Fincham, G.W.; Strauss, C.; Montero-Marin, J.; Cavanagh, K. Effect of breathwork on stress and mental health: A meta-analysis of randomized-controlled trials. *Sci. Rep.* **2023**, *13*, 432. [CrossRef]
58. Ferreira, J.B.; Plentz, R.D.M.; Stein, C.; Casali, K.R.; Arena, R.; Lago, P.D. Inspiratory muscle training reduces blood pressure and sympathetic activity in hypertensive patients: A randomized controlled trial. *Int. J. Cardiol.* **2013**, *166*, 61–67. [CrossRef]

Disclaimer/Publisher's Note: The statements, opinions and data contained in all publications are solely those of the individual author(s) and contributor(s) and not of MDPI and/or the editor(s). MDPI and/or the editor(s) disclaim responsibility for any injury to people or property resulting from any ideas, methods, instructions or products referred to in the content.

MDPI AG
Grosspeteranlage 5
4052 Basel
Switzerland
Tel.: +41 61 683 77 34

Journal of Clinical Medicine Editorial Office
E-mail: jcm@mdpi.com
www.mdpi.com/journal/jcm

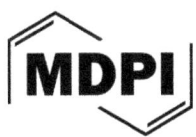

Disclaimer/Publisher's Note: The statements, opinions and data contained in all publications are solely those of the individual author(s) and contributor(s) and not of MDPI and/or the editor(s). MDPI and/or the editor(s) disclaim responsibility for any injury to people or property resulting from any ideas, methods, instructions or products referred to in the content.

www.ingramcontent.com/pod-product-compliance
Lightning Source LLC
LaVergne TN
LVHW070600100526
838202LV00012B/523